OncoLink Patient Guide: Colorectal Cancer 2nd edition

For Elsevier Saunders:
Publisher: Peter Harrison
Development Editor: Kim Benson
Production Manager: Yolanta Motylinska
Design: Kneath Associates

Oncolink Patient Guide: Colorectal Cancer

2nd edition

James M Metz, MD

Editor-in-Chief, OncoLink
Assistant Professor, Department of Radiation Oncology,
University of Pennsylvania, Philadelphia, PA, USA

Margaret K Hampshire, RN, BSN, OCN

Managing Editor, OncoLink
University of Pennsylvania, Philadelphia, PA, USA

ELSEVIER
SAUNDERS

EDINBURGH LONDON NEW YORK OXFORD PHILADELPHIA ST LOUIS
SYDNEY TORONTO 2005

ELSEVIER
SAUNDERS

© 2005, Trustees of the University of Pennsylvania. Published by Elsevier Limited. All rights reserved.

First edition 2003

ISBN 0-7020-2842-8

British Library Cataloguing in Publication Data
A catalogue record for this book is available from the British Library.

Library of Congress Cataloging in Publication Data
A catalog record for this book is available from the Library of Congress.

Note
Medical knowledge is constantly changing. As new information becomes available, changes in treatment, procedures, equipment and the use of drugs become necessary. The author/contributors and the publishers have taken great care to ensure that the information given in this text is accurate and up to date. However, readers are strongly advised to confirm that the information, especially with regard to drug usage, complies with the latest legislation and standards of practice.   *The Publisher*

Working together to grow
libraries in developing countries

www.elsevier.com | www.bookaid.org | www.sabre.org

ELSEVIER   BOOK AID
             International   Sabre Foundation

**your source for books,
journals and multimedia
in the health sciences**

www.elsevierhealth.com

The
publisher's
policy is to use
**paper manufactured
from sustainable forests**

Printed in Canada

CONTENTS

PREFACE

OncoLink (http://www.oncolink.upenn.edu) is one of the oldest and largest cancer information resources on the Internet. OncoLink was developed to provide patients and healthcare providers with the most up-to-date and accurate information on cancer-related issues. Based at the University of Pennsylvania, OncoLink provides a high level of integrity and peer review and has become one of the most trusted resources for cancer information.

OncoLink's content is driven by the needs of its user base. An 'ask the experts' section was established by the editors of OncoLink to address the most important issues of patients and healthcare providers in a timely fashion. OncoLink currently receives hundreds of e-mail questions every week. Numerous experts in the field of oncology answer these questions. This book consists of a compilation of questions regarding colorectal cancer prevention, screening, diagnosis, treatment, and management. Included in this book is a cancer diary for the reader to keep track of important information, including physician contacts, medication lists, and previous treatments. Also, in the appendix section is the National Colorectal Cancer Research Alliance (NCCRA) questionnaire. This was developed for patients interested in becoming involved with colorectal cancer prevention and treatment trials. The questionnaire can be filled out directly online at the OncoLink website, or mailed to OncoLink for entry in the database. The database is regularly searched by NCCRA scientists for patients who match the requirements of new clinical trials and are willing to consider participation.

Please feel free to send comments and questions via e-mail to editors@oncolink.upenn.edu. We hope this book benefits you and your family.

James M Metz, MD

ACKNOWLEDGMENTS

Katrina Claghorn, MS, RD is a registered dietitian at the Abramson Cancer Center at the University of Pennsylvania. Before specializing in oncology Katrina worked in medical nutrition and with patients with eating disorders. Since 1995 she has specialized in oncology nutrition. She now works as an outpatient dietitian in her role as the nutritionist for the Abramson Cancer Center at the University of Pennsylvania. She is also a section editor on nutrition and diet for OncoLink.

Carolyn Coyle, MSN, RN, AOCN is a certified advanced practice oncology nurse. She has worked in the areas of bone marrow transplant, medical oncology, and clinical research. She coordinates OncoLink's collaboration with EmergingMed, a clinical trials matching service for patients. Carolyn manages The National Colorectal Cancer Research Alliance's Clinical Trials Resource Center, assisting callers and managing the NCCRA's clinical trials database. This, along with her nursing experience, has helped her develop a strong knowledge of colon cancer screening, prevention, and treatment. Carolyn writes articles for OncoLink on colon cancer, clinical trials, and human-interest stories.

Bruce Giantonio, MD is an Assistant Professor of Medicine in the Hematology-Oncology division at the University of Pennsylvania. He is also the Executive Officer for the Eastern Cooperative Oncology Group. His clinical expertise lies in the area of colon cancer treatment. His research interests include the use of targeted therapies for gastrointestinal malignancies and new drug development.

Daniel G. Haller, MD is a Professor of Medicine in the Hematology-Oncology division at the University of Pennsylvania. He serves as the Associate Chief for Clinical Affairs and the Co-Program Leader of the Clinical Investigations Program at the Abramson Cancer Center at the University of Pennsylvania. He also holds the position of Editor-in-Chief of the Journal of Clinical Oncology. His clinical expertise is in the area of gastrointestinal cancer, with a special research interest in clinical trials in GI malignancies.

Margaret K Hampshire, RN, BSN, OCN is the Managing Editor of OncoLink and a certified oncology nurse. She has practiced in the areas of gynecologic and surgical oncology. She coordinates all content on the OncoLink website and has a strong interest in cancer-patient education.

Timothy C Hoops, MD is a Clinical Assistant Professor of Medicine in the Gastroenterology Division at the University of Pennsylvania and Director of Gastroenterology at Penn Medicine at Radnor. Dr Hoops specializes in colorectal cancer and is the Director of the Gastrointestinal Cancer Risk Evaluation Program with the University of Pennsylvania. His research interests include colon cancer screening and prevention.

James D Lewis, MD, MSCE is an Assistant Professor of Medicine, Senior Scholar at the Center for Clinical Epidemiology and Biostatistics, and Senior Fellow in the Leonard Davis Institute of Health Economics at the University of Pennsylvania. Dr Lewis specializes in care for patients with inflammatory bowel disease. His research program has focused largely on cancer prevention and the pharmacoepidemiology of gastrointestinal diseases.

Li Liu, MD is a Radiation Oncologist at St Agnes Cancer Center in Fresno, California. He treats a variety of malignancies with radiation therapy. Since completion of his residency at the University of Pennsylvania, he has developed a special interest in the treatment of colorectal cancers.

James M Metz, MD is Editor-in-Chief of OncoLink and Assistant Professor of Radiation Oncology at the Hospital of the University of Pennsylvania. He specializes in the use of radiation for the treatment of gastrointestinal malignancies. His research interests include the clinical applications of photodynamic therapy (PDT), the utilization of complementary and alternative medications by cancer patients, and use of the Internet to provide cancer-related information.

Peter J O'Dwyer, MD is a Professor of Medicine in the Hematology-Oncology division at the University of Pennsylvania. He serves as the Program Leader of the Chemoprevention Program at the Abramson Cancer Center at the University of Pennsylvania. His clinical expertise is in the area of GI cancer, with special expertise in colon/pancreas cancer and new therapies in early clinical trials. His research interests lie in new therapy development for cancer and cancer pharmacologies.

Lora Packel MS, PT is the Coordinator of Cancer Therapy Services for the Hospital of the University of Pennsylvania. Her special area of interest is working with patients after high-dose chemotherapy and/or bone marrow transplantation. She works with head and neck cancer patients before, during, and after treatment, with the ultimate goal of increasing quality of life through exercise.

Anil K Rustgi, MD is an expert in the clinical and genetic aspects of colon cancer. His work is related to basic science research using different models to study the mechanisms underlying the development and progression of colon cancer. In addition, his work involves the discovery of new genes in colon cancer. Dr Rustgi is also devoted to the clinical aspects of inherited colon cancer (familial adenomatous polyposis (FAP) and hereditary non-polyposis colorectal cancer (HNPCC)) and sporadic colon cancer. Ultimately, these efforts are towards improving the screening, diagnosis, and therapy of colon cancer.

Bradley Somer, MD is currently practicing hematology–oncology at the West Clinic in Memphis, Tennessee. Dr Somer's fellowship training took place at the University of Pennsylvania Cancer Center. His internship and residency were also completed in Philadelphia at the Hospital University of Pennsylvania. He has won awards for outstanding scholarship, devotion to patient care, and concern for colleagues.

James P Stevenson, MD is an Assistant Professor of Medicine in the Division of Hematology/Oncology at the University of Pennsylvania. His specialties include thoracic oncology and developmental therapeutics, and his research focus is in early clinical trials of novel agents for the treatment of lung cancer.

Ellen Sweeney-Cordes, MS, RD is a registered dietitian at the Abramson Cancer Center at the University of Pennsylvania. Ellen has worked in several nutrition positions, including inpatient acute care, cardiac nutrition, nutrition in the elderly, and clinical research. She has specialized in oncology nutrition for the past 4 years and currently works with outpatients at the Abramson Cancer Center at the University of Pennsylvania.

Richard Whittington, MD is a Professor of Radiation Oncology at the University of Pennsylvania School of Medicine. Dr Whittington's long-standing interest is in the management of rectal tumors.

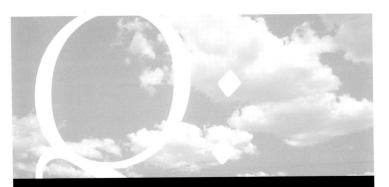

Introduction

NORMAL COLON AND RECTUM FUNCTION

The colon is part of a section of the digestive tract called the large intestine. The large intestine is a tube that is 5–6 feet in length. The first 5 feet make up the colon, which connects to about 6 inches of rectum, and ends with the anus. By the time food reaches the colon (about 3–8 hours after eating) the nutrients have been absorbed and it has become a liquid waste product. The function of the colon is to change this liquid waste into stool. The stool can spend anywhere from 10 hours to several days in the colon. It has been suggested that the longer the stool remains in the colon, the higher the risk for colon cancer, but this has not been proven.

WHAT IS COLON CANCER?

Colon cancer is malignant tissue that grows in the wall of the colon. The majority of tumors begin when normal tissue in the colon wall forms an adenomatous polyp, or precancerous growth projecting from the colon wall. As this polyp grows larger, the tumor is formed. This process can take many years, which allows time for early detection with screening tests.

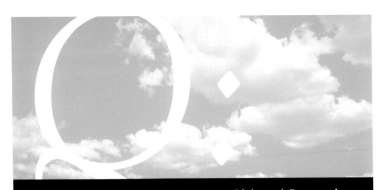

Risk and Prevention

Colon cancer is the third most common type of cancer, in both males and females, in the western world. The incidence is highest in blacks, who are also more likely to die of the disease. Certain factors put people at higher risk, but with over 135,000 new cases each year in the USA, we must all be aware of this deadly disease. The risk of colon cancer rises substantially at age 50, but every year there are numerous cases in younger people. Individuals with a personal or family history of colon cancer or polyps, inherited colon cancer syndromes (i.e. familial adenomatous polyposis (FAP) and hereditary non-polyposis colorectal cancer (HNPCC)), and patients with ulcerative colitis or Crohn's disease are at higher risk, and may require screening at an earlier age than the general population. A person with one first-degree relative (parent, sibling, or child) with colon cancer is 2–3 times as likely to develop the cancer as someone who does not have an affected relative.

However, this does not mean that people without a family history are not at risk. About 80% of new colon cancer cases are diagnosed in people who would not be identified as being at high risk. Studies of colon cancer cases found that lifestyle factors may put a person at higher risk. These factors include: a diet high in fat and red meat, low in fruits and vegetables, high caloric intake, low levels of physical activity, and obesity. In addition, smoking and excessive alcohol intake may play a role in colon cancer development. Despite avoiding all these factors, some people will still develop colon cancer. With screening and early detection, these patients can be cured in the majority of cases.

Polyps. Ten years ago I had polyps. They were not cancerous. Could they become cancerous?

Regarding polyps, some can become cancerous. However, if your polyps were completely removed, you are unlikely to develop cancer.

Importantly, even if your polyps were removed, you could develop new polyps. You should speak with your primary care physician about colon cancer surveillance. ■

James D Lewis, MD, MSCE

66
if your polyps were completely removed, you are unlikely to develop cancer

Colon cancer can present with many different symptoms. Among these are:

- abdominal pain

- a change in your bowel habits (e.g. new constipation)

- weight loss

- rectal bleeding

- blood in the stool (on the stool, in the toilet bowl, or on the tissue paper)

- persistent abdominal cramps

- chronic diarrhea or constipation

- unusual fatigue.

Importantly, some patients with colon cancer may have no symptoms at all. This is why regular screening and communication with your doctor is so important. ■

James D Lewis, MD, MSCE

> 66
> Colon cancer can present with many different symptoms, but some patients with colon cancer have no symptoms at all

Rectal bleeding and flat stools. Sometimes after a bowel movement, I notice blood on the tissue paper and a streak of blood along one side of the flat stool. What is the significance of this finding?

Blood visible in the stool can be caused by non-cancerous (benign) problems, such as hemorrhoids, diverticulitis, colitis, or tears in the skin due to forcing a bowel movement when constipated. However, this can also be a sign of colon or rectal cancer. The fact that you can see the blood implies that the source of bleeding is close to the rectum. When bleeding is present further up the gastrointestinal tract it is not visible, but may turn stools a darker (black or tar) color. This bleeding can be detected by a fecal occult blood test, which can be performed by your doctor. In this test, a small amount of stool is placed on a special card, and then a solution (called developer) is applied to the card. The card turns blue if blood is present in the stool. Although this bleeding may seem harmless, it is worth investigating with your doctor.

You also mentioned that your stools have a flat appearance, which is concerning. Changes in the shape of stool can be another sign of colon or rectal cancer. As a tumor grows in the colon or rectum, it can change the shape of the bowel that the stool passes through. This may cause stools to become thinner, pencil like or flat in shape. You should report these problems to your physician for further investigation. ■

Carolyn Coyle, MSN, RN, AOCN

"
blood visible in the stool and a change in shape of the stool can be signs of colon or rectal cancer

It has long been suggested that a low frequency of bowel movement, by increasing concentrations of cancer-causing agents (carcinogens) in the stool and increasing their time of contact with the gut wall, elevates the risk of colorectal cancer. In the USA, where colorectal cancer is the third highest cause of cancer death, 15–20% of adults are reported to suffer from constipation. A similar proportion of adults report regular use of laxatives. Previous epidemiologic studies on constipation and cancer have shown inconsistent results, in part because of the complexity in characterizing bowel movements. The widespread use of laxatives further complicates the relationship between the frequency of bowel movement and the risk of colorectal cancer. Recently, phenolphthalein, the active ingredient in many laxative brands, has been shown in animal feeding studies to cause several different tumors, although not colorectal cancer.

People may be able to lower their risk of developing colorectal cancer by managing the factors that they can control, such as diet and physical activity. It is important to eat plenty of fruits, vegetables, and whole-grain foods and to limit intake of high-fat foods. Physical activity is another area that people can control. Even small amounts of exercise on a regular basis can be helpful. ■

Li Liu, MD

66

It is important to eat plenty of fruits, vegetables, and whole-grain foods and to limit intake of high-fat foods

There is no reason to believe that hemorrhoids lead to colorectal cancer. However, the symptoms of hemorrhoids are often similar to those of colorectal cancer or anal cancer. Some symptoms of hemorrhoids include:

- rectal bleeding

- blood in the stool

- blood on the stool

- blood in the toilet bowl

- blood on the tissue paper.

As such, it is important to see your doctor to have these symptoms evaluated. If you are concerned about any of these symptoms you should see your physician for an examination. ■

James D Lewis, MD, MSCE

> 66 There is no reason to believe that hemorrhoids lead to colorectal cancer

Hereditary colon cancer. *I have an intensive family history of colon cancer. My paternal grandfather died from it in his 50s. My father has had seven colon polyps removed and his two sisters have had colon cancer recently. I also have had three colon polyps removed and have ongoing abdominal pain and bloating at times. I am currently seeing my physician for this. What information is available on hereditary connections for colon cancer?*

Based on your description, it appears that your family may have a form of familial colon cancer called hereditary non-polyposis colorectal cancer (HNPCC). It is defined by clinical and genetic criteria. The clinical criteria include three or more family members with colon cancer; one should be first-degree relative of the other two, spanning two generations and one case before age of 50. These criteria have been modified recently to take into account variants of HNPCC and genetic understanding.

Often it is recommended for HNPCC-associated families that the siblings, father, and paternal aunts (and their children) have a periodic colonoscopy (every 1–2 years).

Endometrial and ovarian cancer can be associated with HNPCC, and therefore women at risk or affected would benefit from an annual pelvic ultrasound scan and, possibly, periodic endometrial biopsies.

Genetically, it is very helpful to obtain tissue blocks from parental aunts for immunohistochemical staining of MSH2, MLH1, and PCR analysis for

"
it appears that your family may have
a form of familial colon cancer called
hereditary non-polyposis colorectal
cancer (HNPCC)

microsatellite instability. Tissue blocks are wax-embedded pieces of tissue that are typically removed during surgery or autopsy. They are saved by the pathology laboratory that first examined them. Often the laboratory saves them for years, and they may be obtained at your request.

Based on these results, it may be recommended that you see a genetic counselor and have MSH2/MLH1 gene testing initially of aunts and then other family members based on the gene testing. ■

Anil K Rustgi, MD

Q: *Prognostic factors including genes. Following surgery for stage B colon cancer last year, at age 64, I elected not to have chemotherapy. I understand that the presence or absence of some genes makes a significant difference in the effectiveness of therapies such as radiation and chemotherapy. Is there a current test to determine whether these genes are present in an individual?*

There are some genes that can be tested for in colon-cancer surgery specimens that may provide information regarding prognosis and predict response to treatment. Two of the genes currently under investigation are called DCC and p53. There is conflicting data regarding the use of p53 to predict response to therapy and overall prognosis. Early studies show that DCC may be an important marker in evaluating patients in the future, but intensive investigation continues. The DCC and p53 genes are not routinely evaluated in surgical specimens and such evaluation would need to be done by a specialized laboratory.

The most important factor regarding prognosis is the presence or absence of cancer in lymph nodes from the surgical specimen. For example, although we cannot comment on your specific case, assuming that the staging information you have presented is correct and complete, Dukes' B colon cancers (no lymph node involvement) have a very good prognosis. We know that most people with node-negative cancers do not benefit

" DCC and p53 genes are not routinely evaluated in surgical specimens and such evaluation would need to be done by a specialized laboratory

from postoperative chemotherapy, so a decision not to have chemotherapy after surgery is a reasonable one.

Current recommendations are continued and close follow-up with an oncologist or surgeon (every 3 months), with blood work (including a CEA test) performed at each visit, as well as follow-up colonoscopies. ■

James P Stevenson, MD

Q: Family history and risk. I am a 31-year-old male. Both grandparents on my father's side were diagnosed with colon cancer at age 50–55. My paternal great grandfather was diagnosed at age 75. Mom has no colon cancer history. So far my father and his four siblings (aged 45–55) are free of the disease and free of polyps. I had a flexible sigmoidoscopy at age 29, which was clear. Would this constitute a possible or likely 'familial' situation?

The lifetime risk of colon cancer is increased for first-degree (parents, siblings, and children) relatives and, to a lesser extent, for second-degree relatives (grandparents, aunts, and uncles). Thus, you are at somewhat increased risk, although it is good that your father and aunts and uncles have yet to manifest polyps or cancer. You should have a screening colonoscopy at some point, and if that is normal your gastroenterologist can determine the frequency of future colonoscopies. ■

Anil Rustgi, MD

66 The lifetime risk of colon cancer is increased for first-degree (parents, siblings, and children) relatives and, to a lesser extent, for second-degree relatives (grandparents, aunts, and uncles)

Q: Irritable bowel syndrome and colorectal cancer.
I am a 33-year-old woman and have been diagnosed with irritable bowel syndrome. Can this condition lead to colorectal cancer?

While some of the symptoms of irritable bowel syndrome may also be symptoms suggesting the presence of a cancer (e.g. a change in bowel habits, constipation), there is no known relationship between irritable bowel syndrome and colon cancer. However, should a cancer develop in a patient with this syndrome it would very likely be caught early, since colonoscopies are often performed to make sure that other problems are not the cause of the symptoms. ■

Timothy C Hoops, MD

66
there is no known relationship between irritable bowel syndrome and colon cancer

Q: *Ulcerative colitis. My mother suffered from ulcerative colitis from age 33 to 42. She finally had a j-pouch surgery and is doing well. Her brother and sister also both have ulcerative colitis and were both diagnosed in their 30s. On my father's side, his father died of colon cancer at age 70, his sister has ulcerative colitis, and he has had polyps removed from his colon. His other sister also has irritable bowel syndrome (which I understand is not related). I am already trying to increase my fiber intake, but it is very difficult for me to get 25 g a day. What else can I do to protect myself and prevent colon problems?*

First of all, while we know that a family history of colon cancer and having ulcerative colitis can each increase a person's risk for colon cancer (and together there may be an additive effect), your risk as an unaffected family member is harder to determine. Your father's history of polyps and your grandfather's colon cancer may raise your lifetime risk, but probably by about two-fold at most. Ulcerative colitis can have a genetic component to it and you may be at risk for developing it, but there is no way to determine this beforehand with any certainty.

66

factors that have been shown to reduce colon cancer risk include calcium, folate (400 mg/day), and exercise. Hormone replacement therapy in postmenopausal women may also be beneficial. The most important thing to do is undergo colon cancer screening

From a preventive standpoint, there is little that can be done for the ulcerative colitis that I am aware of. For colon cancer, there is no strong evidence that fiber decreases the risk, although there are other beneficial effects of fiber that might warrant its use. Other factors that have been shown to reduce colon cancer risk include calcium, folate (400 mg/day), and exercise. Hormone replacement therapy in postmenopausal women may also be beneficial. The most important thing to do is undergo colon cancer screening. Unless you have symptoms, you can probably wait until you turn 50. At a minimum, this should be annual stool occult blood testing (Hemoccult) and a flexible sigmoidoscopy every 5 years, or a colonoscopy every 10 years. This is the best colon cancer risk reduction method available. ■

Timothy C Hoops, MD

Q: *Lynch syndrome. I have just learned that a lot of our family members are carriers of Lynch syndrome. I am told it is a form of colon cancer. What more can you tell us?*

Lynch syndrome is one of the inherited syndromes that is characterized by a high risk for the development of colon cancer. Several abnormal genes have been discovered as the culprits for this disease. It is a dominantly inherited syndrome, meaning that if the abnormal gene is inherited from the parent, the person will have the disease (see p. 29). If a parent has the disease, there is a 50% chance that they will pass it on to their children. If the parent does not have the disease, it cannot be passed on to the next generation (i.e. it does not appear to skip generations).

There are other cancers that can occur in Lynch syndrome, most notably uterine and ovarian cancer in women. The goal in patients who are at risk is to try to prevent these cancers. As such, routine colonoscopic screening examinations are recommended. OncoLink has joined forces with the National Colorectal Cancer Research Alliance to help their scientists study the risk factors associated with colorectal cancer and identify potential preventive and treatment therapies. You and your family may be interested in taking part in our survey. This confidential survey was developed by cancer experts as an interactive way to help our leading scientists study families with a history of colorectal cancer. Please fill out the survey located at the end of this book. ■

Timothy C Hoops, MD

> ❝ Lynch syndrome is one of the inherited syndromes that is characterized by a high risk for the development of colon cancer

Is colon cancer hereditary? I have just been diagnosed with a Dukes' B adenocarcinoma of the colon, which has now been removed, and I am about to start a course of chemotherapy (5-FU). I am only 26 years old and have been told it is very unusual for someone of my age to get bowel cancer and that there is most likely a genetic cause. Can you explain how this happens?

Colon cancer is very unusual in people under 50 years old, but it can and does occur in younger people. In many cases this is related to the inheritance of one of several genes that predispose that person to colon cancer. Since the cancer is related to these genes, other members of the family are usually also affected with colon cancer or other related cancers.

You make no mention of any family history in your case. If there is a family history, it may be worth exploring that possibility. If there is no family history of cancer, it is still possible that your cancer could be related to a gene defect. Presumably, this would be due to a new mutation. Some have suggested that anyone with an early-onset colon cancer should be tested for genetic mutations, regardless of family history. The advantages of doing this would be to get a better understanding of what led to the disease, to increase awareness of other possible associated tumors and to know what the risks are for transmission of the cancer susceptibility to children (if a mutation were found, the children could also be tested as they grew older).

66

the inheritance of one of several genes
predisposes a person to colon cancer

It is important to understand, however, that the chance of finding a genetic mutation is still relatively small. The important thing for anyone with colon cancer is that, after the treatment phase, an active surveillance program is necessary, given the risk for the development of new cancers. In addition, any first-degree relatives should also undergo a colonoscopy, as they are also at a significantly increased risk for colon cancer. ■

Timothy C Hoops, MD

Q:

Symptoms of colon cancer. I have abdominal discomfort, bloating, gas, constipation, nausea, and pencil-thin stools. I am 44 years old, female and have no medical insurance. What can I do to find out if I have cancer or what the problem is?

The symptoms you describe are non-specific and could possibly be due to any number of things, including parasites, inflammatory bowel disease, irritable bowel syndrome and cancer. This list is far from complete. The good news is that the longer you go without a diagnosis, the less likely that your symptoms are due to cancer, as this disease progresses unless treated. Without insurance, I would agree that it might be difficult to get the work-up you need. Maybe you can check with your local department of social services to see if they have an assistance or Medicaid program available for you. Universities and large hospitals often have clinics that will accept patients without insurance. You may be able to work out some type of payment program with your physician to get some of this work done.

Your symptoms sound very bothersome and, regardless of whether they are from cancer or not, they should be evaluated and treated. ■

Timothy C Hoops, MD

" Universities and large hospitals often have clinics that will accept patients without insurance

Colorectal cancer accounts for 14% of all cancer deaths in the USA. There were an estimated 135,400 new cases and 56,700 deaths in the USA in 2001. Approximately 10–15% of these cancers may be caused by genetic abnormalities that run in families. There are two major types of known hereditary disorders: familial adenomatous polyposis (also known as FAP) and hereditary non-polyposis colorectal cancer (also known as HNPCC). Here we will address FAP.

FAP accounts for only 1% of new colorectal cancer cases each year, affecting about 1 in 9,000 people. About 15% of people with FAP develop polyps by the age of 10, and 90% develop them by the age of 30. Affected patients can develop hundreds to thousands of adenomatous polyps, and have a 100% chance of developing colorectal cancer by age of 40 if they do not have their colon removed. Adenomatous polyps are considered to be 'precancerous' lesions, some of which will eventually progress to cancer. Therefore, the more polyps an individual has, the greater his or her chance of developing cancer. The average age of colorectal cancer diagnosis in FAP is 35 years, as compared to 64 years in the general population.

Several other cancers have been associated with FAP, including periampullary and thyroid cancer. Periampullary cancer (cancer that is found in the area where the bile duct and pancreas empty into the small bowel) is the second most common cancer in FAP, and accounts for 1 in 5

" FAP accounts for only 1% of new colorectal cancer cases each year, affecting about 1 in 9,000 people

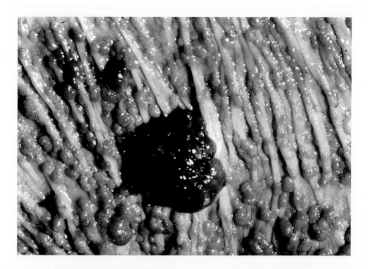

Colon with multiple adenomas. Photo courtesy of the Familial GI Cancer Registry, Toronto, Canada.

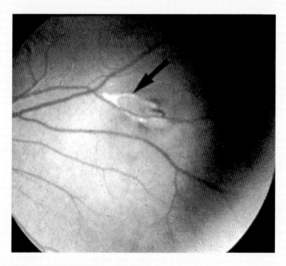

Congenital hypertrophy of the retinal pigment epithelium. Photo courtesy of the Familial GI Cancer Registry, Toronto, Canada.

deaths of these patients. In addition, several other non-cancerous manifestations have been seen in FAP. Young FAP patients may develop cysts in the skin on the face, scalp, arms, and legs, often years before they develop colon polyps. Congenital hypertrophy of the retinal pigment epithelium (also called CHRPE) is an abnormality found in the retina of the eye that looks like a freckle and causes no symptoms for the patient. While CHRPE can be seen in one eye of individuals without FAP, it is often present in both eyes in an FAP patient. About 70% of FAP patients have dental abnormalities, including extra or missing teeth, fused roots, or non-cancerous tumors of the jaw bone (osteomas). Although these manifestations are not harmful to the patient, they may be the first sign of FAP and prompt a patient to undergo testing for FAP. Ten percent of FAP patients will develop desmoid tumors, which are non-cancerous, slow-growing tumors that occur in the abdominal area. Despite the fact that these tumors are not cancerous, they can cause significant damage by surrounding, compressing, and eroding nearby structures, and may need to be removed surgically. In the past, the term 'Gardner's syndrome' was used to describe a subset of FAP patients that have CHRPE, dental abnormalities or desmoid tumors, and was thought to be genetically different. It is now known that these features are seen in many FAP patients and these cases are not genetically different.

GENETICS AND SCREENING

In 1991, the gene responsible for FAP was discovered and was named the adenomatous polyposis coli, or APC, gene. Scientists have discovered over 300 different mutations in the APC gene which can cause FAP. The location of the mutation on the gene often correlates with the number of polyps, age of onset, and other manifestations. FAP is an autosomal dominant inherited disorder, meaning that a child of an affected parent has a 50% chance of inheriting the mutation. Approximately 30% of FAP cases are 'de novo mutations', meaning that there is no prior family history of the mutation.

The diagnosis of FAP is made by discovering >100 adenomatous polyps or through genetic testing in a known FAP family. Once a person has been diagnosed with FAP, an analysis of the family should be done to determine the likelihood that other relatives have the condition. Genetic testing can identify the specific abnormality in the affected individual, and then look for this defect in other family members. It is recommended that children of FAP patients undergo genetic testing or endoscopic screening by the age of 10. If genetic tests are positive in these children, endoscopic screening should be done every 1–2 years. If genetic testing is negative, these people can be spared the intensive screening.

Genetic testing is something that should not be taken lightly. One must consider the affect of the test results on the individual and their family members. Concerns may include the implication of a positive or negative test, passing the gene on to children, and discrimination in employment and insurance matters. A genetic counselor should meet with anyone wishing to undergo testing, both before testing and after the results are known. These professionals are trained to help patients understand the risks and benefits of testing and what to do with the results.

TREATMENT

There is no medication to prevent the development of colon polyps in FAP, but non-steroidal anti-inflammatory drugs (NSAIDs), such as sulindac and indomethacin, have been shown to shrink polyps in these patients. Clinical trials are currently examining ways to prevent polyp growth in these patients. Until better medical therapies have been developed, these patients require surgical removal of the colon (colectomy) to prevent the development of colon cancer. This surgery is often performed between the ages of 17 and 20 in asymptomatic members of FAP families. There are several surgical options for these patients, but the goal is to remove all colorectal tissue at risk for developing polyps and maintain normal bowel evacuation through the anus.

FAP is one of the most well-understood inherited cancer syndromes. This knowledge has led to the availability of genetic testing for at-risk individuals, improved screening and surgical management, and clinical trials for the prevention of polyp formation. Continued research into FAP will lead to better treatments for these families, and may have implications for all colon cancer patients. ■

Carolyn Coyle, MSN, RN, AOCN

Hereditary non-polyposis colon cancer. I have a number of relatives who have developed colon cancer over the years. I was recently informed that my family has a syndrome called HNPCC and we should all be screened with a colonoscopy. Can you tell me more about this diagnosis?

Colorectal cancers are some of the most common cancers in industrialized countries. In 2001, there were an estimated 135,400 new cases and 56,700 deaths in the USA. Approximately 10–15% of cases may be caused by genetic abnormalities that run in families. There are two major types of hereditary disorders that lead to colorectal cancers: familial adenomatous polyposis (also known as FAP) and hereditary non-polyposis colorectal cancer (HNPCC). HNPCC accounts for about 5–10% of all colorectal cancers, while FAP cases make up only about 1%.

Dr Henry Lynch first described HNPCC, and the disorder is often referred to as 'Lynch syndrome' (see p. 21). He further specified that families either had Lynch type I (also called HNPCC type A) or Lynch type II (also called HNPCC type B). Families with Lynch type I often report numerous cases of colorectal cancers in young (age <50 years) relatives. The average age of diagnosis of cancer in patients with this syndrome is 44 years, as compared to 64 years in people without the syndrome (which is often referred to as a 'sporadic cancer'). Families with the Lynch type II syndrome will also report colorectal cancers in young relatives, but will also have cases of 'HNPCC-related cancers'. These related cancers include cancer of the breast, endometrium, gastrointestinal system, ovaries, and ureter.

" specific criteria must be met and certain genetic abnormalities must be present for a family to be classified as HNPCC

Although many patients may have similar family histories, specific criteria must be met and certain genetic abnormalities must be present for a family to be classified as HNPCC. The genes that have been identified as responsible for HNPCC are MSH1, MSH2, PMS1, and PMS2. Individuals with a mutation in any one of these genes have an estimated 80% lifetime risk of developing colon cancer. People with HNPCC are most likely to develop cancer on the right side of the colon, unlike most sporadic cases, which develop on the left side of the colon. Flexible sigmoidoscopy, a standard screening test for colorectal cancer, only examines the left side of the colon, and is a poor screening test for this population. While people with HNPCC develop polyps at the same rate as other people, these polyps are more likely to progress to cancer. In addition, the progression of polyps to cancer occurs in a shorter period of time compared to sporadic cases of colorectal cancer.

In order to better define families with HNPCC, a panel of experts met in 1990 in Amsterdam to develop criteria for the syndrome, often referred to as the 'Amsterdam criteria'. In the years following this meeting, genetic testing became more readily available and a number of families have been found to carry one of the genetic abnormalities, but do not fit the original criteria. For this reason, in 1999 the Amsterdam criteria II were developed, and these now serve as the necessary criteria for HNPCC families.

The criteria are:

- There should be at least three relatives with an HNPCC-associated cancer (colorectal, endometrial, small bowel, ureter, or ovarian).

- One should be a first-degree relative of the other two (a first-degree relative is a parent, sibling, or child).

- At least two successive generations should be affected.

- At least one relative should be diagnosed before the age of 50.

- FAP must be ruled out, and the tumors must be verified by pathology.

Families with histories meeting the criteria may wish to undergo genetic testing to determine if they carry the defective gene. If this test (usually done on the affected family member's tumor) is positive for a genetic abnormality, other family members at risk can then be tested for the same abnormality. If no abnormality is detected in the family member's tumor, then testing other family members would not be informative. However, the tests that are currently available are not 100% accurate. Depending on the methods used, they can miss positive cases anywhere from 5% to 50% of the time. A family may carry a mutation in a gene that has not yet been discovered or a mutation for which that testing has not yet been developed.

Genetic testing is something that should not be taken lightly. One must consider the effect of the outcome of the test not only on themselves, but also on other family members. Concerns may include the availability, or lack of, preventive options, passing the gene on to one's children, and discrimination in employment and insurance matters. To assist in this difficult decision, a genetic counselor should meet with anyone wishing to undergo testing. These professionals are trained to help patients understand the issues surrounding genetic testing, and help them make the right decision for them and their family.

People with HNPCC tend to develop cancers earlier than the general population, and therefore should begin screening earlier. It is estimated that 15% of people with HNPCC will develop colorectal cancer by age 40. People with HNPCC should have a colonoscopy, beginning at age 20–25 years, and repeated every 1–2 years. Women in these families are at increased risk for endometrial cancer, and should consider annual transvaginal ultrasound or endometrial biopsy starting at age 25–35.

Scientists have learned a great deal about genetic syndromes in the past 10 years. This is, in part, due to the involvement of patients in research studies. ■

Carolyn Coyle, MSN, RN, AOCN

The most important step one can take to minimize their risk of either developing or dying of colon cancer is to enroll in a colon cancer screening program. Screening can be performed by testing stool for the presence of blood or by visualizing all or a portion of your colon either with x-rays or with endoscopy. Early detection and removal of precancerous polyps can dramatically reduce the risk of developing colon cancer. Some clinical trials on the prevention of colon cancer are currently under way. ■

James D Lewis, MD, MSCE

> ❝ The most important step one can take to minimize their risk of either developing or dying from colon cancer is to enroll in a colon cancer screening program

Use of aspirin probably reduces the risk of developing colon cancer, but it does not entirely eliminate the risk. Therefore, even if you are taking aspirin, you should still participate in a colon cancer screening program. A number of trials have been developed or are under design to prevent the development of colorectal cancer. Please consider enrollment in the OncoLink/National Colorectal Cancer Research Alliance colorectal cancer prevention database (see the end of this book), and register if you are interested in exploring clinical trials evaluating these new agents. ∎

James D Lewis, MD, MSCE

66 Use of aspirin probably reduces the risk of developing colon cancer, but it does not entirely eliminate the risk

There has been a great deal of research on the impact of nutrition on colon cancer. Despite all the studies there is still no definitive anti-colon cancer diet. Below is a list of nutritional factors that have been found to have the greatest potential for reducing colon cancer risk.

■ A high intake of dietary fat, especially saturated fats mostly found in animal sources, has been shown to increase the incidence of colon cancer. Red meat in particular has been associated with increasing risk. Include more fish, poultry and low-fat dairy products in your diet.

■ Fiber was long considered an important preventive factor, but the results of recent research have been conflicting. It is still wise to strive for at least 25 g/day of fiber for general good health.

■ High levels of calcium have been associated with decreased polyp formation. While dietary sources of calcium are encouraged, calcium supplements have also been found to be beneficial.

■ Folic acid acts to prevent damage to DNA, which can trigger the cancer process. While folic acid is found in dark green vegetables and dried beans and legumes, it is now added to enriched breads and cereals.

■ Some studies indicate that the antioxidant vitamins A, C, and E, as well as the mineral selenium, may reduce the incidence of colon

" Despite all the studies there is still no definitive anti-colon cancer diet

cancer. While the benefits of taking supplements of these nutrients are still being debated, adding more fruits and vegetables to your diet is advised.

- Obesity is associated with increased risk of developing colon cancer. Try to maintain a healthy weight.

- Regular exercise has been found to be protective.

Katrina Claghorn, MS, RD

The risk of developing colon cancer in persons with Crohn's disease is related to the extent of colon that is involved by the Crohn's disease. Patients with only small bowel Crohn's disease (i.e. no disease in the colon) appear to have a risk of colon cancer comparable to that in the general population. In contrast, patients with extensive Crohn's disease of the colon appear to have a substantially increased risk of colon cancer. These patients should be followed rigorously by their gastrointestinal specialist, with frequent screening evaluations. Please see the OncoLink/National Colorectal Cancer Research Alliance colorectal cancer prevention survey at the end of this book, and register to be considered for colorectal cancer prevention trials. ■

James D Lewis, MD, MSCE

> " The risk of developing colon cancer in persons with Crohn's disease is related to the extent of colon that is involved by the Crohn's disease

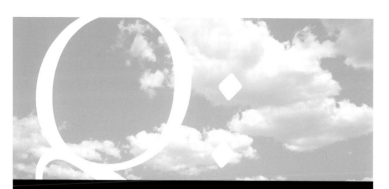

Screening and Diagnosis

Colon cancer screening tests. I am at high risk for colon cancer because my mother had colon cancer at age 37, my maternal great aunt had colon cancer, and my father's mother died of colon cancer. How often should I have a colonoscopy?

According to the American Cancer Society and the American Gastroenterological Association colorectal cancer screening guidelines, men and women over the age of 50 and not in a high-risk group (see below) should use the following guidelines:

■ yearly fecal occult blood test plus flexible sigmoidoscopy every 5 years,* or

■ colonoscopy every 10 years,* or

■ barium enema every 5–10 years.*

People are considered at high risk for colon cancer when they have any of the following risk factors:

■ a strong family history of colorectal cancer or polyps (cancer or polyps in a first-degree relative younger than 60 or in two first-degree relatives of any age)

*A digital rectal examination (DRE) should be performed at the time of each screening sigmoidoscopy, colonoscopy, or barium enema examination.

❝ yearly fecal occult blood test plus flexible sigmoidoscopy every 5 years, or colonoscopy every 10 years, or barium enema every 5–10 years.

- families with hereditary colorectal cancer syndromes (familial adenomatous polyposis and hereditary non-polyposis colon cancer)

- a personal history of colorectal cancer or adenomatous polyps

- a personal history of chronic inflammatory bowel disease.

For those in a high-risk group, especially those with a family history of colorectal cancer, the American Cancer Society and the American Gastroenterological Association recommend the above screenings at age 40 and a colonoscopy every 3–5 years thereafter. ■

Li Liu, MD

CEA as a screening tool. If the CEA (carcinoembryonic antigen) blood test is done to determine if cancer has returned in a patient, then why can't this test be done first? Could the CEA blood test be used as a screening test for colon cancer?

Your question, and the concept you are proposing, is excellent and has been the Holy Grail of cancer screening. A simple blood test that would reliably identify patients with early cancers and rule out those who do not have cancer would be the perfect screening exam. Unfortunately, no such test exists. CEA is a protein that is found in several tissues, but in particular, it is in the colon. With cancer, this protein can be made in increased amounts and shed into blood. It has been carefully studied as a screening test. Unfortunately, the test is not very sensitive. The amount of CEA protein in the blood is frequently normal and thus the test would miss cancers. In addition, other factors, such as smoking, can raise the CEA level. The test is used in patients who have had cancers resected to look for recurrences, with the hope that these will be found early enough to treat successfully. Even in this case, the test is generally useful only when the initial cancer was CEA positive and the levels returned to normal after the initial treatment.

Ongoing research into other markers for cancer continues. Whoever finds such a test will have given us a great way to decrease the impact of and number of deaths from colon cancer. ■

Timothy C Hoops, MD

66
The amount of CEA protein in the blood is frequently normal and thus the test would miss cancers

Guidelines for colon cancer screening. I am a 26-year-old female. Both my mother and grandmother developed colon cancer, at the ages of 49 and 55, respectively. At what age should I have a colonoscopy?

It is not possible to provide an answer specific for you without knowing more details of your family's medical history. The current guidelines for persons with a family history of colorectal cancer would be to begin screening around age 40. However, with two relatives on your mother's side having colorectal cancer, and one before age 50, it is possible that you should be screened earlier. You should seek consultation with a gastroenterologist and ask them this question. By providing more detailed information about your family history, they can provide you with better guidance. You might consider joining the OncoLink/National Colorectal Cancer Research Alliance colorectal cancer prevention database (see the end of this book). ■

James D Lewis, MD, MSCE

> " The current guidelines for persons with a family history of colorectal cancer would be to begin screening around age 40

Q: Frequency of screening colonoscopy. I have a history of colon cancer on both sides of my family. My previous doctor recommended having a colonoscopy every 2 years. I recently moved and my new doctor recommends every 5 years. How often should I have a colonoscopy?

There are no absolute guidelines for the frequency of colonoscopy when one is doing them for average risk screening. In the USA, Medicare has just released guidelines stating that they will reimburse for screening colonoscopies every 10 years. A flexible sigmoidoscopy has been recommended every 4–5 years and some physicians have extrapolated this to colonoscopies.

For people with an increased risk for cancer, the guidelines are clearer. For those with a history of colonic polyps, colonoscopy should be performed every 3–5 years, based on the findings of the last colonoscopy. For those with a history of colon cancer, a repeat procedure should be done at 1 year and, if negative, at either 2 or 3 years after that. If the procedures show no new polyps or cancers, the interval can safely be stretched to 3–5 years. Patients with a family history of colon cancer should have a colonoscopy every 5 years if they have no polyps and every 3 years if they do.

Please understand that, while some of these recommendations are based on studies designed to answer these questions, some of the recommendations are based on expert opinion with indirect data for support. Your physician should determine the appropriate interval for your screening procedures based on your results. ■

Timothy C Hoops, MD

66
Patients with a family history of colon cancer should have a colonoscopy every 5 years if they have no polyps and every 3 years if they do

Colonoscopy after polyp removal. My father underwent a colonoscopy at age 70. Polyps were removed. How often should he have a colonoscopy?

In the early 1990s a study was done in which about 1500 patients who had undergone polypectomy were divided randomly into two groups. One group had follow-up colonoscopies at 1 and 3 years. The other group had a repeat colonoscopy at 3 years only. The study demonstrated that there was no difference between the two groups in the number of recurrent polyps or cancers found. This changed the practice of gastroenterology from yearly follow-up colonoscopy, which had been the standard, to every 3 years.

The same researchers have shown that if there were fewer than three polyps and they were very small, it was probably safe to even wait 5 years for the next procedure. These data support what is known about the biology of the development of cancer. In most, if not all, cases cancers develop from adenomatous polyps. The process of going from normal tissue to polyp to cancer is quite long, extending from 10 to 15 years and possibly even longer. Thus, the longer interval between colonoscopies after removal of a polyp is safe and reduces the discomfort and small risk associated with this procedure.

It may benefit your father to have a colonoscopy no sooner than 3 years, unless there was some specific finding that warranted an earlier procedure. ∎

Timothy C Hoops, MD

66
It may benefit your father to have a colonoscopy no sooner than 3 years, unless there was some specific finding that warranted an earlier procedure

Screening options when insurance companies refuse to pre-certify a colonoscopy. I have had alternating constipation and diarrhea for about 2 years, with constricted stools and bloating. It has steadily gotten worse over the last 6 months. My physician referred me to a gastroenterologist to have a colonoscopy. My insurance company will not pre-certify a colonoscopy. They want me to have a sigmoid first, then maybe a colonoscopy. Both my parents, my grandmother, and many aunts and uncles have died of other cancers. What should I do?

If you are over 50 years old, you should be able to argue for a colonoscopy as a screening procedure. Even if you are over 40, you might be able to push that argument. You have had a change in bowel habits, and that may warrant some type of procedure. If you are young, a flexible sigmoidoscopy may be sufficient. As you stated, you may have to show that it is negative before a colonoscopy is approved.

You also mentioned a family history of cancer, but not of the colon. There are not many sporadic cancers that are associated with colon cancer, so I would not be too concerned about that unless it appears that you might have one of the inherited cancer syndromes. I would recommend that you go back to your internist or gastroenterologist and ask what they feel the

66
You have had a change in bowel habits, and that may warrant some type of procedure

best test would be. If it is a colonoscopy, I would be persistent with your insurance company. The 'squeaky wheel' often does get the grease, but you must persist. Unfortunately, healthcare decisions are not always left to the patient and the physician. ■

Timothy C Hoops, MD

Insurance coverage for colonoscopy. My brother is 58 years old and has never had a colonoscopy. My mother had breast cancer that metastasized to her colon, requiring a colostomy. My father has recently been diagnosed with colon cancer, detected on a colonoscopy. The physician told my brother that he should have a colonoscopy immediately. The insurance company is denying payment for the colonoscopy and have said they will pay for it only if there is 'active bleeding'. At 58 years old and with such a strong family history, my brother obviously needs the colonoscopy, and his primary care physician (PCP) agreed, or he would not have referred him in the first place. What should he do in this situation?

Coverage of colonoscopies by insurance companies has become an increasingly larger problem. Many companies are now covering 'screening' colonoscopies for patients who are not above average risk for the disease. The rationale is that this procedure is more complete. It may also be safe to do this procedure once every 10 years. People such as your brother, who have a family history of colon cancer, have an increased risk for the development of colon cancer, reaching 10–15% over their lifetime. Most gastroenterologists would recommend a full colonoscopy for these patients, as the entire colon can be evaluated and if polyps are found they

66
Coverage of colonoscopies by insurance companies has become an increasingly larger problem

can be removed. Alternative recommended screening methods include a flexible sigmoidoscopy every 5 years and annual tests for occult blood in the stool. The opinion of many experts is that this may be a somewhat less effective method for screening patients with an increased risk for colon cancer.

Unfortunately, healthcare insurers use many criteria to determine how they cover certain services. Discussion of the specific issues regarding risk may cause them to change their policy for an individual. It should be stressed that any symptom such as a change in bowel habits or any rectal bleeding can then be used as a justification for the procedure. Finally, it is our hope that these policies will be changing in the near future as more public support is generated for better screening techniques. ■

Timothy C Hoops, MD

Q: *Risks of colonoscopy. I am in the process of looking for a qualified professional to perform my first colonoscopy. I spoke with a doctor and she informed me that she has had three experiences where perforations took place and one person actually died. I am apprehensive about having her perform my colonoscopy. Is my concern well founded? What credentials should I ask for as I look for a doctor to perform this?*

I would agree that you should have a colonoscopy as you are at much higher risk than the general population for colon cancer. I also understand your concern about the risks of the procedure. In all the hub-bub about screening colonoscopies that has been presented in the press, this issue is often overlooked.

In general, the risk of perforation during colonoscopy is very small. The medical literature suggests a risk of between 1 in 500 and 1 in 10,000. Suffice it to say that your risk for cancer is significantly greater, although still small. Your doctor was particularly open and straightforward with you; many are not so detailed. That does not imply lesser skills. One would have to know the number of procedures she has performed and the aspects of the individual cases, as there are numerous things that may have predisposed to perforations. The risk in a healthy young person is very small.

> make sure your physician has been formally trained to perform colonoscopies in an accredited program, has performed a large number of them (preferably at least several hundred), and is board certified by their specialty

As to credentials, I would make sure your physician has been formally trained to perform colonoscopies in an accredited program, has performed a large number of them (preferably at least several hundred), and is board certified by their specialty. You should feel confident that your physician is fully capable of doing the procedure and, in the unfortunate event of a complication, is able to recognize and deal with the situation.

To summarize, while you should be aware that there are complications with colonoscopy, as there are with any medical intervention, there are also risks of not having the procedure. These risks generally outweigh those of the procedure. ■

Timothy C Hoops, MD

Virtual colonoscopy is currently being developed. It is a series of ultrathin computed tomography (CT) scan images that are stacked by a computer and then the large intestine is isolated. The procedure is currently investigational, as the early data from a few centers have suggested that it may be nearly as effective in their hands as conventional colonoscopy. It is time consuming, since it may involve imaging 100–250 CT slices, and the images need to be manipulated after they have been obtained. In institutions that do these studies, the patients currently undergo conventional colonoscopy as well to determine the accuracy of the virtual study. All the centers involved in the study have shown that there is a very steep learning curve. The test is least sensitive in detecting villous adenomas, and these are the polyps most likely to contain cancers. It is still necessary to take the bowel prep, and this needs to be more effective than is needed for colonoscopy. Also, due to its experimental nature, insurance companies may not currently reimburse the cost of the procedure. ■

Richard Whittington, MD

66
a series of ultrathin computed tomography (CT) scan images that are stacked by a computer and then the large intestine is isolated

Carcinoembryonic antigen, or CEA, is a glycoprotein that is present in many tissues, including the cells that line the colon. Since colon cancers develop from these cells, one can find elevated CEA levels in the blood of patients who have colon cancer. The CEA level can also rise with other cancers.

The most common use for measuring CEA levels is to look for recurrence of colon cancer after treatment. If there is an elevated CEA prior to surgery, it will usually return to normal if the entire tumor has been removed. Subsequent monitoring may signal a recurrence of the cancer. The CEA test has been promoted as a way to detect a recurrence before it is clinically apparent, allowing earlier and, hopefully, more effective re-treatment. Unfortunately, some colon cancers do not present with elevated CEA levels, which makes it a less than perfect test.

The other proposed use of the CEA level is to screen for colon cancer. Unfortunately, levels are uncommonly elevated, especially with small early cancers, resulting in a high false-negative rate. In addition, the CEA level can be mildly elevated in smokers or in other cancers, resulting in a high false-positive rate. Between these false-positive and false-negative tests, it is too unreliable as a test to screen for colon cancer. ■

Timothy C Hoops, MD

> The most common use for measuring CEA levels is to look for recurrence of colon cancer after treatment

Q:
CEA and the OncoScint scan. What is the validity
and usage of the CEA test, and how reliable is the
OncoScint scan when looking for current disease?

Carcinoembryonic antigen (CEA) is one of the oncofetal proteins, which is at its highest normal levels during embryonic or fetal life and may re-arise with some malignancies, such as breast, colorectal, pancreatic, lung, and ovarian cancer. Non-malignant diseases that may cause elevation of CEA include cirrhosis, chronic obstructive pulmonary disease, and smoking. Following treatment for colorectal cancer, serial CEA measurement is thought to be the most sensitive laboratory test for recurrent cancer. However, the potential therapeutic benefit of postoperative CEA monitoring remains controversial due to potential costs and questionable long-term effectiveness.

Given your history of stage III rectal cancer in 1996, a rising CEA level is very concerning. The exact cause of the elevation may never be determined, but steps to rule out recurrent rectal cancer would be appropriate. The OncoScint and CEA Scan were developed a few years ago and are currently available for the detection of colorectal carcinoma, especially recurrent disease. OncoScint uses indium-111 labeled B72.3, which is a murine monoclonal antibody to bind Tag-72. Tag-72 is a cell-surface antigen, which is expressed by colorectal carcinoma cells. The CEA scan uses a technetium-99m labeled fragment of the anti-CEA antibody for the detection of pelvic recurrence of colorectal carcinoma. Both methods have been used in addition to the conventional diagnostic methods, including computed tomography (CT)

" The accuracy of OncoScint is about 70%, based on early clinical experience scan and magnetic resonance imaging (MRI). However, the exact roles of these two immunoscintigraphic studies remain controversial and need to be defined. The accuracy of OncoScint is about 70%, based on early clinical experience. Exploratory laparotomy is often required to obtain a definitive diagnosis and resect the recurrent disease whenever feasible. ■

Li Liu, MD

A polyp is a growth in the colon. There are several types of polyps. Some are referred to as 'adenomatous polyps'. These are considered to be precancerous, meaning that, given enough time, most would progress to cancer. Others are not precancerous, meaning that they probably have little or no risk of becoming a cancer. Importantly, we know that removal of precancerous polyps dramatically reduces the chances that a person will develop colon cancer. ■

James D Lewis, MD, MSCE

> " removal of precancerous polyps dramatically reduces the chances that a person will develop colon cancer

Villous adenoma. I am a 38-year-old woman who recently had a villous adenoma removed and remnants cauterized. There was also a small polyp removed. I had the adenoma cauterized again a few months later and I am going back for another evaluation soon. My mother died of breast cancer. My father had polyps. Will the villous adenoma ever come back or does cauterization kill it at the site? What caused it, since I have no risk factors?

How often should it be checked? Am I at risk for more of these villous adenomas at other sites or colon cancer? The cells on top had changed. My doctor said it would be cancer in a year if not removed, but the cells underneath were OK. What behavior modification can I do? I eat pretty healthily.

If your polyp was completely removed, it should not recur

Although we understand some of the reasons polyps and colon cancer develop, we often are surprised and feel that it is all random and fortuitous. If your polyp was completely removed, it should not recur. The issue with a larger polyp is whether it has been removed completely. I assume that is the reason why you have had several follow-up colonoscopies. When you are completely clear, you can probably have a colonoscopy every 3 years. Once you have had a couple of clear colonoscopies without polyps, you may be able to expand the interval to 5 years.

You are already doing most of the behavioral preventive strategies. You might want to add a vitamin with at least 400 µg/day folic acid. Although there is some evidence that drugs such as aspirin and some of the other pain medications may help prevent colon cancer, there still is not good enough evidence to routinely recommend this. However, it is something you and your physician could discuss. It is not clear whether the risks outweigh the benefits. You do have an increased risk with your father's history of colon polyps. Your mother's history of breast cancer may play some role, but that is not clear. As with any disease, there will always be people who develop a disease despite doing all the right things.

OncoLink has joined forces with the National Colorectal Cancer Research Alliance to help their scientists study the risk factors associated with colorectal cancer and identify potential preventive and treatment therapies. You and your family may be interested in taking our survey. This confidential survey was developed by cancer experts as an interactive way to help our leading scientists study families with a history of colorectal cancer. Please see the end of this book for information on enrollment in this database. ■

Timothy C Hoops, MD

An intramucosal carcinoma of the colon is a pathological diagnosis. In general, these are cancerous cells that are out of their normal location, but have moved only slightly into the surrounding tissue. If this truly was the finding, then the odds are strongly in your favor that this has been completely removed and should cause no further problem. There should be no problem if you want to get a second pathology opinion to confirm the findings. This is obviously a very early cancer. As such, the chance for a cure with a polypectomy is nearly complete, although one cannot be 100% certain. It is usually recommended that a follow-up colonoscopy be done within about 6 months to be certain that the entire polyp has been removed. Thereafter, you should get another study done in about 3 years to look for new polyps. Your doctor should be able to tailor the follow-up recommendations to fit your particular situation.

I would agree that you are a good example of why one should undergo colon cancer screening. If you had not, there is an excellent chance you would have progressed to a more advanced colon cancer with less of a chance for a cure. ■

Timothy C Hoops, MD

> 66 In general, these are cancerous cells that are out of their normal location, but have moved only slightly into the surrounding tissue

Q: *Virtual colonoscopy and DNA stool testing.* I have heard about some new screening tests for colon cancer called a virtual colonoscopy and DNA stool testing. Can I avoid a regular colonoscopy if I have these tests?

In 2001 in the USA there were an estimated 135,400 new cases of colon cancer and 56,700 deaths due to the disease. When detected early, colon cancer can be cured in 90% of cases. However, only 44% of adults over the age of 50 undergo screening tests for colon cancer. Current screening tests include fecal occult blood testing, flexible sigmoidoscopy, and colonoscopy. The low rate of testing may be due to one of several factors: apprehension about the tests, the preparation before the test, or fear of what may be discovered. Whatever the reason, the reluctance to undergo screening only worsens the situation.

In the past 2 years, there has been widespread media coverage of potential alternatives to the traditional methods of screening for colon cancer. It seems that people see these tests as a way to potentially avoid colonoscopy or sigmoidoscopy. In order for new methods to replace traditional testing, they need to be as effective, similar in cost, and be accepted by patients.

VIRTUAL COLONOSCOPY

Virtual colonoscopy, a method of viewing the colon from outside the body, employs the use of a computed tomography (CT) scan. Throughout the procedure, the patient lies on a table that passes through a 'donut'-like

" Currently, the virtual test does not perform as well as its conventional counterpart

machine that takes pictures from different angles around the body. The two-dimensional images of the colon are converted by a computer to three-dimensional images, and then reviewed by a trained radiologist. This is quite time consuming, requiring approximately 30 minutes per patient, which adds to the cost of the procedure. In order for these images to be accurate, patients must undergo a bowel prep similar to that for traditional colonoscopy, but for the virtual scan the bowel needs to be clearer. For the bowel prep, patients take laxatives and modify their diet for up to 24 hours before the procedure. Just prior to the CT scan, a tube is inserted into the rectum and air is pumped into the colon allowing it to expand. This allows better visualization of the bowel wall. Patients are also given an intravenous medication called glucagon, causing the bowel walls to relax, which also improves visualization of the colon.

The accuracy of virtual colonoscopy varies greatly with the training of the radiologist who is interpreting the scan. Currently, the virtual test does not perform as well as its conventional counterpart. This may change as the procedure is refined and radiologists become better trained. Studies have found that virtual colonoscopy is not as accurate in detecting flat or smaller lesions (<5 mm). Some physicians have suggested that the smaller polyps are less likely to progress to cancer, and therefore the decreased ability to detect them may not be significant, but this has not yet been proven.

Two studies have evaluated patient preferences regarding the tests by measuring discomfort, feelings of disrespect or embarrassment, and which test they would rather have. Both studies found that patients preferred conventional colonoscopy in all three categories. In both studies, patients received sedation for the conventional colonoscopy, but not for the virtual test, which is standard, but may have an effect on patient preferences. It is important to consider that virtual colonoscopy is a diagnostic procedure, and if a polyp is detected the patient would then need to undergo conventional colonoscopy to remove the polyp. Some suggest that this be done on the same day to avoid the need for a second bowel prep, but this may be unrealistic in busy medical centers.

At this time virtual colonoscopy is not widely available and is mostly done as part of a clinical trial, in which patients undergo both procedures for comparison. Because it is still considered experimental, insurance companies do not currently cover this procedure. Many advances have been made in virtual colonoscopy in just a few years, and the technique will continue to improve. However, the issues of cost-effectiveness, accuracy, and patient preference will need to be addressed before this test can become a standard of care.

DNA STOOL TESTING

In DNA stool testing, scientists examine stool for genetic abnormalities that are found in colon cancer. A patient's stool sample is analyzed using polymerase chain reaction (PCR) testing to determine whether mutations in the adenomatous polyposis coli (APC) gene are present. One study, recently reported in *The New England Journal of Medicine*, analyzed samples from 28 patients with early stage (Dukes' B2) colon cancers, 18 from patients with adenomas (cancerous polyp) of at least 1 cm, and samples from 28 patients without cancer. The test was able to detect mutations in 26 of the 46 patients with cancer (57% of the cases detected). The researchers reported that no gene abnormalities were detected in the 28 patients without cancer. DNA stool testing, with a 57% detection rate, would be unacceptable as a replacement for current screening methods, but this study paves the way for more research into this testing method.

Given the current low utilization rates of colon cancer screening in adults, there is obviously a need for increased education and the development of less invasive, more acceptable, yet accurate methods of screening. Virtual colonoscopy and DNA stool testing are promising, and we are sure to hear more about them in the coming years, but for now, schedule your sigmoidoscopy or colonoscopy! ▪

Carolyn Coyle, MSN, RN, AOCN

" DNA stool testing, with a 57% detection rate, would be unacceptable as a replacement for current screening methods

After a cancer has been found, the stage must be determined to decide on appropriate treatment. The stage tells how far the tumor has invaded the colon wall, and if it has spread to other parts of the body.

- Stage 0 (also called carcinoma in situ): the cancer is confined to the outermost portion of the colon wall.

- Stage I (also called Dukes' A colon cancer): the cancer has spread to the second and third layers of the colon wall, but not to the outer colon wall or beyond.

- Stage II (also called Dukes' B colon cancer): the cancer has spread through the colon wall, but has not invaded any lymph nodes (these are small structures that help in fighting infection and disease).

- Stage III (also called Dukes' C colon cancer): the cancer has spread through the colon wall and into lymph nodes, but has not spread to other areas of the body.

- Stage IV (also called Dukes' D colon cancer): the cancer has spread to other areas of the body (i.e. liver and lungs).

After the tumor and lymph nodes have been removed by a surgeon, they are examined by a pathologist, who determines how much of the colon wall and lymph nodes have been invaded by tumor. Patients with invasive cancer (stages II, III, and IV) require a staging work-up, including

66 The stage tells how far the tumor has invaded the colon wall, and if it has spread to other parts of the body

full colonoscopy, carcinoembryonic antigen (CEA) level (a marker for colon cancer found in the blood), chest x-ray, and computed tomography (CT) scan of the abdomen and pelvis, to determine if the cancer has spread. ■

Carolyn Coyle, MSN, RN, AOCN

Fecal occult blood testing, also known as FOBT, is a test that can detect blood in the stool, even when it is not visible to the eye. This test involves placing a small amount of stool on a special card. A solution (or developer) is then applied to the card, and the card turns blue if blood is present. This test can be done at your doctor's office, or at home, and brought to the doctor's office for developing. Polyps or colon and rectal tumors may cause intermittent bleeding, and FOBT may be able to detect this bleeding, prompting further testing. It is important to note that some foods may cause the test to be positive. Ask your physician what foods to avoid when doing this test. The American Cancer Society recommends that this test be done every year, in conjunction with a sigmoidoscopy every 5 years. ■

Carolyn Coyle, MSN, RN, AOCN

66
FOBT is a test that can detect blood in the stool, even when it is not visible to the eye

Sigmoidoscopy is a procedure that utilizes a sigmoidoscope to examine the rectum and the first portion of the colon. It is important to note that this procedure does not evaluate the entire colon. The sigmoidoscope is a long, slender, flexible tube that contains a light and a camera. When inserted into the rectum, the bowel wall can be visualized with the camera, and projected onto a television screen that the doctor can see. In order to see the bowel wall, the patient must undergo a bowel preparation the day before the test. This may include a laxative, enema, and a clear liquid diet. The American Cancer Society recommends that people over 50 years old have this test every 5 years, or a colonoscopy every 10 years. ■

Carolyn Coyle, MSN, RN, AOCN

" a procedure that utilizes a sigmoidoscope to examine the rectum and the first portion of the colon

Q: *Digital rectal examination. What is a digital rectal examination?*

A digital rectal examination is a technique used by physicians to assess rectal function, feel for rectal tumors or hemorrhoids, and check for blood in the stool. The physician inserts a finger into the patients' rectum and is able to feel the first few inches of the rectal tissue. By obtaining a small amount of stool, the fecal occult blood test can then be used to check for blood in the stool. In men, this test can also be used to evaluate the prostate gland. ■

Carolyn Coyle, MSN, RN, AOCN

" technique used by physicians to assess rectal function, feel for rectal tumors or hemorrhoids, and check for blood in the stool

A barium enema uses barium sulfate, a radio-opaque contrast material that allows the bowel to be viewed using an x-ray. The test requires a bowel preparation the day before the procedure, which may include a laxative, enema, and clear liquid diet, to rid the colon of any stool. The barium is infused through a tube in the rectum, into the colon. The patient is placed on a table that moves in various directions in order to fully visualize the colon while the x-rays are taken. This test can be used to diagnose tumors, bowel obstruction, and other abnormalities including ulcerative colitis. ■

Carolyn Coyle, MSN, RN, AOCN

66
This test can be used to diagnose tumors, bowel obstruction, and other abnormalities including ulcerative colitis

Endoscopic ultrasound was first used in the early 1980s. It essentially involves the use of a scope (slender, flexible tube) that has an ultrasound scanner on the end of it. Ultrasound technology uses sound waves of extremely high frequency to allow the physician to 'see' through the colon wall. This helps determine the depth of the tumor and if any nearby lymph nodes are enlarged, suggesting that tumor has spread to them. It can be used for staging in any gastrointestinal tumor, including colon, gastric, esophageal, and pancreatic cancers. ■

Carolyn Coyle, MSN, RN, AOCN

66
sound waves of extremely high
frequency allow the physician to 'see'
through the colon wall

Colonoscopy is a procedure that utilizes a colonoscope to examine the rectum and entire colon. The colonoscope is a long, slender, flexible tube that has a light and a camera, which allows the bowel wall to be seen by the physician on a television screen. In addition, the colonoscope contains instruments that allow the doctor to take samples of tissue from the bowel wall when necessary. The colonoscope can be used to view the whole colon, unlike the sigmoidoscope with which only about half of the colon can be seen. The patient must undergo a bowel preparation the day before the procedure, and this needs to be more complete than the preparation for sigmoidoscopy. This preparation may include laxatives, enemas, and a clear-liquid diet. The American Cancer Society recommends that people without a family history of colon cancer have this test every 10 years for screening, or a sigmoidoscopy every 5 years. ■

Carolyn Coyle, MSN, RN, AOCN

66

a procedure that utilizes a colonoscope to examine the rectum and entire colon

Anemia is a condition where the oxygen-carrying component in the blood (called hemoglobin) is low. Anemia can be caused by a deficiency in a substance necessary to produce blood (iron-deficiency anemia), inherited abnormalities (sickle-cell anemia), problems with the bone marrow (leukemia, aplastic anemia), or the body's own destruction of red blood cells (hemolytic anemia). Chronic illnesses can also cause a person to be anemic (e.g., cancer, rheumatoid arthritis).

Chronic blood loss can also make a patient anemic. Gastrointestinal bleeding is a common source of chronic blood loss. Colon or rectal cancers can cause this type of bleeding. As it grows, a colon or rectal tumor invades the wall of the bowel, causing it to bleed slowly. Over time, this blood loss can lead to anemia. To test for this type of bleeding, your doctor may perform a fecal occult blood test, which tests to see if blood, not visible to the eye, is present in the stool. If this test is positive, the patient needs to undergo a test to examine the colon for abnormalities.

A colonoscopy is a test that allows the physician to examine the entire colon for any cause of bleeding. If a polyp is found it can be removed during the procedure. A sigmoidoscopy only examines part of the colon, and in a patient with symptoms there is the concern that something significant in the rest of the colon may be missed. Colorectal cancer is the third most common cancer in both men and women. Although most commonly occurring in people over age 50, thousands of cases are diagnosed every year in younger people. Although family history may

66 a colon or rectal tumor invades the wall of the bowel, causing it to bleed slowly

play a part in the decision to screen, 80% of new cases are diagnosed in people with no family history of the disease. It is recommended that all people over age 50 undergo screening for colon cancer, regardless of whether or not symptoms are present. ■

Carolyn Coyle, MSN, RN, AOCN

When a polyp is removed during a colonoscopy it is sent to a pathologist for review. The doctor may have removed all that was visible, but this needs to be confirmed microscopically. The pathologist examines the polyp under a microscope to be sure that all the polyp cells were removed. This report will also tell if the polyp was cancerous or not. As long as the entire polyp was removed, there is nothing to do right away.

It is likely that patients who have polyps at one time will form new ones in the future. Polyps grow very slowly, thus allowing time for them to be detected before they become cancerous. Not all polyps will become cancerous, but we cannot predict which will and which will not, so all polyps should be removed. After a polyp has been found and removed, the patient should have a colonoscopy every 3–5 years. This will allow future polyps to be detected before they can become cancerous. ■

Carolyn Coyle, MSN, RN, AOCN

> " Polyps grow very slowly, thus allowing time for them to be detected before they become cancerous

Testing after a positive sigmoidoscopy. A cancerous polyp was found on sigmoidoscopy. Do I need other tests?

Any patient who has a positive sigmoidoscopy needs follow-up testing with colonoscopy. If polyps were present in the lower third of the colon (the section evaluated by sigmoidoscopy), there may be polyps in other areas of the colon. The polyps must also be removed, which may not have been done with the sigmoidoscope. Once removed, a pathologist examines the polyps. The pathology report tells whether the polyp is cancerous or not, if the entire polyp was removed, or if cells were left behind. This report dictates whether or not further treatment is needed. ■

Carolyn Coyle, MSN, RN, AOCN

" Any patient who has a positive sigmoidoscopy needs follow-up testing with colonoscopy

If a polyp was found, it was presumably removed and examined by a pathologist. The pathologist's report will tell if the polyp is cancerous or not, if the entire polyp was removed, or if any cancerous cells were left behind. If the pathology report shows that cancerous cells may have been left behind, surgery may be necessary to remove the bowel around this area and nearby lymph nodes for examination.

It is likely that patients who have polyps at one time will form new ones in the future. Polyps grow very slowly, thus allowing time for them to be detected before they become cancerous. Not all polyps will become cancerous, but we cannot predict which will and which will not, so all polyps should be removed. After a polyp has been found and removed, the patient should have a colonoscopy every 3–5 years. This will allow future polyps to be detected before they can become cancerous. ∎

Carolyn Coyle, MSN, RN, AOCN

" If the pathology report shows that cancerous cells may have been left behind, surgery may be necessary

Colon cancers are classified by microscopic descriptions of their cells. The most common type is adenocarcinoma, which makes up 90–95% of all colon cancers. The three types of adenocarcinoma are mucinous adenocarcinoma, signet-ring adenocarcinoma, and adenosquamous carcinoma, which is a mix of two types. Rarer types of colon cancer include: squamous carcinoma, small-cell carcinoma, choriocarcinoma, and medullary carcinoma. On rare occasions, two other types of tumors, carcinoid and sarcoma, may present in the colon. The different types of colon tumors are treated differently, based on their cell type. Most of the information available for patients on the treatment of colon tumors is for adenocarcinomas. ■

Carolyn Coyle, MSN, RN, AOCN

66 different types of colon tumors are treated differently, based on their cell type

Biopsy of a colon polyp. I had a biopsy of a colon polyp. What does the pathologist look for and why does it take so long?

The pathologist's report is very important, and often dictates the plan for treatment. The specimen is sent to a laboratory, which may be outside the hospital or doctor's office where the biopsy was performed. The specimen is split into smaller samples to allow better viewing under the microscope. The specimen is then examined carefully to see that the entire polyp has been removed. This is done by looking for normal tissue around the polyp, referred to as 'clear margins', meaning the specimen's margins are free of abnormal cells. If the margins are not clear, further surgery may be necessary to remove the abnormal tissue left behind. The pathologist reports the cell type, which tells if the polyp is cancerous or not. If the polyp is cancerous, the cell type will help plan further treatment. In the case of a bowel resection, the pathologist also examines the lymph nodes to look for tumor cells.

The examination by the pathologist can take some time, as it includes evaluation of both the visible specimen and a microscopic evaluation. Each specimen needs to be carefully prepared, sectioned appropriately, and placed in special stains for defined periods of time. Only after these procedures have been carried out can the pathologist carefully review each slide (of which there may be many) under the microscope. The final pathology report will include gross (visible inspection) and microscopic (cellular) analysis. ■

Carolyn Coyle, MSN, RN, AOCN

> 66
> The specimen is examined carefully to see that the entire polyp has been removed

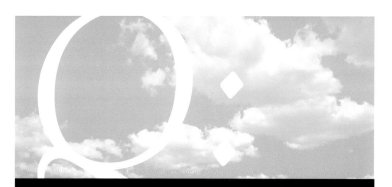

Stage I colon cancer is a tumor that has begun to invade the wall of the colon. This tumor is removed surgically and requires no further treatment. These patients should receive follow-up surveillance with colonoscopy, but carcinoembryonic antigen (CEA) testing, computed tomography (CT) scans, or x-rays are not warranted.

In stage II and III colon cancers, the tumor has deeply invaded the bowel wall, or grown through the wall, and can involve nearby organs. In both cases, surgical removal of the tumor, a section of the bowel surrounding the tumor, and local lymph nodes for pathologic evaluation is required. The differentiation between the two stages is made by the examination of the lymph nodes. In stage II colon cancer there is no cancer present in the lymph nodes, whereas in stage III colon cancer there is. In addition, as part of the staging work-up, these patients should have a full colonoscopy (to look for other polyps or tumors), CEA testing, CT scan of the abdomen and pelvis, and a chest x-ray.

The treatment of stage II colon cancer is somewhat controversial. Most studies of postoperative chemotherapy (called adjuvant chemotherapy) for stage II colon cancer have failed to show any improvement in patient survival. Despite these results, it is generally agreed that there is a subset of higher risk stage II patients who probably would benefit from adjuvant chemotherapy. High-risk patients include those who present with bowel obstruction, perforation, or tumor involvement of other organs. These patients may be eligible to participate in a clinical trial evaluating adjuvant chemotherapy in this population. In general, these patients would be treated with a regimen of 5-FU (5-fluorouracil) and leucovorin for 6 months.

The treatment of stage III colon cancer is better defined and has been validated by many studies. These patients are treated for 6 months with a 5-FU and leucovorin regimen, of which there are several variations. The regimen may be chosen based on physician preference or the ability of the patient to tolerate the side-effects of that regimen.

Radiation therapy in colon cancer has limited use. Patients who have residual tumor after surgery, invasion of another organ, or an adhesion (an area where the tumor has stuck to the abdominal wall) may benefit from radiation treatment to that area.

Stage IV colon cancer has spread to other organs (e.g. liver, lung). A patient may be diagnosed originally at this stage, or have progressed from stage II or III. Either way, the treatments are generally not for cure, but to improve quality of life and extend the patient's survival.

Surgery in stage IV disease varies from case to case, and is not always performed. The stage may not be discovered until after surgery has been performed, or part of the colon may be removed to provide relief from symptoms caused by the cancer. In some cases it may be more important to start systemic treatment with chemotherapy, rather than to perform surgery and have to allow time for healing before starting drug treatment. In the case of progressive disease, the surgery may have been done months to years previously.

Chemotherapy for patients who are in generally good health (also known as a good performance status) can improve quality of life and may extend survival by a few months. Chemotherapy in patients with a poor performance status has not shown much benefit, and may worsen quality of life. The standard regimen for stage IV disease in the USA is 5-FU, leucovorin, and irinotecan (CPT-11 or Camptosar). This has been shown to be superior to the combination of 5-FU and leucovorin in these patients. Studies are still evaluating the effectiveness of adding irinotecan to the regimen for stage III disease.

Two other agents, capecitabine (Xeloda) and oxaliplatin, are being used in patients with advanced colon cancer where other treatment has failed or where the patient is unable to tolerate standard therapy. Xeloda is an oral form of 5-FU, and may be better tolerated by patients, although it is not without side-effects. Oxaliplatin is widely used in Europe, and has just been approved for use in the USA.

- *Can both procedures be done at the same time?*

- *Is there a risk of spreading the cancer to the 'open' wound where the diverticula are removed?*

- *How will I know if I need radiation and/or chemotherapy?*

- *How long will the surgery keep me out of work?*

- *What questions should I be asking the surgeon?*

- *What questions should I be asking my gastroenterologist?*

- *How do you choose the right guy and the right place?*

First, your gastroenterologist and your surgeon are the best ones to answer these questions, as they know the most details about the extent of your disease and that information will determine the course of your therapy.

> **"** meet with and 'interview' the doctors before anything further is done

Finding the right physician may be hard, but you can ask your friends and other physicians for their opinions. You should meet with and 'interview' the doctors before anything further is done. The most important things are that the physicians are experienced and you are comfortable with them. If not, choose another doctor. Sometimes a person with a great reputation may be worth having despite their 'bedside manner', but remember that they have to take care of you.

Two colonic resections can be done simultaneously, if necessary. It makes the operation longer, but should not put you at risk for spread of the cancer, if done correctly.

Whether you need further therapy such as chemotherapy or radiation therapy will be determined by the extent of the cancer as determined by the pathologist after your surgery. If the cancer has spread outside the colon, your oncologist will probably recommend treatment (adjuvant chemotherapy).

The recovery period varies from one person to another. In the usual case, you will probably be in the hospital for about 1 week. Your recovery time before returning to work may be 6 weeks, but that will depend on the type of work you do as well as your individual progress. ■

Timothy C Hoops, MD

You do not always need a colostomy for the treatment of colon cancer. In fact this has become less and less common as surgical methods have improved over the years. Surgery is the most common treatment for colon cancer. If the cancer is limited to a polyp, the patient can undergo a polypectomy (removal of the polyp), or a local excision, where a small amount of surrounding tissue is also removed. If the tumor invades the bowel wall or surrounding tissues, the patient will require a partial resection of the bowel (removal of the cancer and a portion of the bowel) and removal of local lymph nodes to determine if the cancer has spread into them. After the tumor has been removed, the two ends of the remaining colon are reconnected, allowing normal bowel function. In some situations, it may not be possible to reconnect the colon, and a colostomy is necessary. A colostomy is when the surgeon passes the end of the colon through the abdominal wall and connects it to the outside of the abdomen, creating an outlet for stool to pass through. Equipment, known as 'appliances', are attached to the abdominal wall to collect the stool.

There are times when a colostomy is necessary temporarily. After the patient has had some treatment with chemotherapy and radiation, the surgeon may be able to reverse the colostomy by reconnecting the bowel ends. Whether or not a patient has a temporary, permanent, or no colostomy at all is determined by the size and location of the tumor, which the surgeon evaluates by means of computed tomography (CT) scan and during surgery. ■

Carolyn Coyle MSN, RN, AOCN

> 66 Whether or not a patient has a temporary, permanent, or no colostomy at all is determined by the size and location of the tumor

Low-anterior resection (LAR) and abdominal perineal resection (APR). What is the difference between low-anterior resection and abdominal perineal resection?

There are important differences between these two types of surgery. An LAR, a low-anterior resection, is done through the abdomen. In this procedure a portion of the rectum is removed and the remaining rectum is sewn to the end of the colon. This may heal slowly and the surgeon may create a temporary colostomy further upstream to rest the newly sewn intestine and allow it to heal. A temporary colostomy is created when the surgeon is concerned that fecal material may leak into the pelvis. This is less of a problem when the surgery is higher up in the abdomen because the pressures in the intestine are not as high as they are in the rectum. A temporary diverting colostomy may also be recommended after radiation or removal of an abscess or in inflammatory bowel disease, as these may contribute to slow wound healing. These temporary colostomies may be closed by sewing the two ends together after 6 weeks to 6 months.

An APR, an abdominal perineal resection, involves an incision in the abdomen as well as a second incision around the rectum. The lower colon and the entire rectum is removed including the sphincter muscles. This requires a permanent colostomy. This procedure is recommended when there is not enough normal rectum left near the anal region to reconnect the bowel. This procedure is not as bad as people think. There are many famous people who have lived for decades with a colostomy and have continued to lead otherwise normal lives. ■

Richard Whittington, MD

> " An LAR, a low-anterior resection, is done through the abdomen
>
> An APR, an abdominal perineal resection, involves an incision in the abdomen as well as a second incision around the rectum

Q:

Removal of tumors and spread to other parts of the body. Can you remove a colon tumor after it has spread to other parts of the body? What is considered inoperable and why?

You can remove a colon tumor after it has spread if the physicians think the patient would benefit. This would include surgery to remove the tumor in order to prevent or relieve obstruction, to control or prevent bleeding, to prevent or alleviate pain, or if there was a concern about infection or invasion of the abdominal wall or skin. Sometimes single metastases are removed surgically in the liver or lung if there is no evidence of other disease spread.

Tumors are considered inoperable when it is thought that surgery will not help. This includes patients who are sick and would not survive an operation, patients in whom the tumor has spread but the tumor is not threatening to cause problems, and patients in whom the tumor is stuck to or invaded by something critical (e.g. blood vessels or organs) and the surgeon cannot get around it safely or effectively. ■

Richard Whittington, MD

66
Tumors are considered inoperable when it is thought that surgery will not help

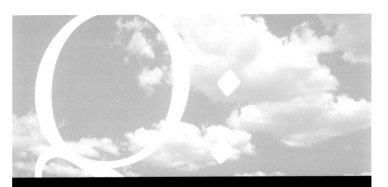

Treatment – Chemotherapy

Erbitux treatment and side effects. My dad has metastatic colon cancer. He was treated last year with irinotecan. Now the doctors say that the cancer is back and he needs to switch to a new drug. They are suggesting Erbitux. They say it works differently than other drugs. Can you explain this treatment and maybe the side-effects my dad can expect? They say it can cause a rash.

Irinotecan is standard first-line therapy for metastatic colon cancer. Over the past year, there have been some new therapies approved in the United States. Cetuximab (Erbitux) has been approved for exactly this setting in combination with irinotecan. Even though your father received irinotecan previously, there can still be significant response when it is given together with cetuximab this time around. Cetuximab is part of a new generation of drugs that are called 'targeted therapies.' It is an antibody that targets something called the epidermal growth factor receptor (EGFR), which is expressed significantly in colon tumors. It is also expressed in normal skin, so a rash can be seen as a side-effect. In fact, it has been shown that those patients who have a rash from the medication also have their tumors respond better to the treatment. Other new therapies that may be considered if your father's tumor does not respond to this regimen are oxaliplatin, which is a newer chemotherapy drug, or bevacizumab, which is a targeted therapy against the substances that stimulate tumor blood vessel formation. ■

Peter J. O'Dwyer, MD

> Cetuximab is part of a new generation of drugs that are called 'targeted therapies'

Q: *Treatment and follow-up options after colon cancer. My wife underwent a colon resection to remove a cancerous growth. One lymph node tested positive. Subsequent chemotherapy treatment (5-fluorouracil and leucovorin) was administered over a 6-month period. What are the follow-up testing procedures? What are the follow-up treatment procedures? What preventive measures are recommended?*

To review: Your wife had a colon resection and there was one node with tumor. Presuming that there is no further evidence of disease or metastases and that the surgeon was able to remove the tumor with adequate margins in its entirety, your wife was given adjuvant chemotherapy (for no current detectable disease, but rather to prevent relapse from the risk of micrometastases). This would most likely be considered a Duke's stage C or a stage III (American Joint Committee on Cancer) colon cancer.

Resection alone is curative in 50% of patients with colon cancer. After resection, adjuvant chemotherapy is given in situations where patients are more likely to relapse. The intention is to prevent future recurrence of disease. Patients with lymph node involvement are candidates for this therapy. Patients with colon cancer with other higher risk features, such as perforation, obstruction, aggressive pathological features, and invasion of any internal organs, are potential candidates for adjuvant chemotherapy. The main data on adjuvant chemotherapy in this setting are from patients with lymph node involvement (stage III).

" Resection alone is curative in 50% of patients with colon cancer

There have been multiple major clinical trials, including those from the Intergroup, National Surgical Adjuvant Breast and Bowel Project, and the North Central Cancer Treatment Group showing significant benefit from adjuvant chemotherapy. In general, the extra benefit obtained from chemotherapy is 22–30% for stage III patients. Standard therapy is with 5-fluorouracil in combination with levamisole or leucovorin. This is the mainstay of preventive strategies for recurrence. Other therapeutic adjuvant chemotherapy strategies are under investigation.

After therapy, patients are typically followed closely to ensure that, should the cancer recur, it is discovered early, thus improving the ability to manage it effectively. Some of the aspects and timing of the studies required during the follow-up are controversial. The National Comprehensive Cancer Network has published guidelines, and the following are adapted from these:

■ Every 3 months for 2 years, then every 6 months for 5 years:

  – Medical history, focusing on weight loss, weakness, loss of appetite, constipation, nausea, vomiting, fevers, and abdominal pain.

  – Physical examination, focusing on weight, lymph node evaluation, abdominal bloating, tenderness, masses, liver enlargement, rectal masses, or stool for occult blood testing.

  – Blood counts.

■ CEA (carcinoembryonic antigen) test, every 6 months for 2 years, then annually for 5 years, but only if the level was elevated prior to or just after surgery. If by following the CEA level the patient does relapse, they would be a candidate for surgical resection of discovered localized recurrence or isolated metastasis.

■ Chest x-ray: for stage B2 or C disease, every 12 months for 5 years.

■ Abdominal computed tomography (CT) scan, approximately every 6 months for 2 years, then annually for 3 years.

■ Colonoscopy within the first year, repeated 1 year later and every 3 years after that if negative for multiple synchronous polyps or if the patient has a new polyp on surveillance colonoscopy.

These recommendations remain controversial, and we recommend following a surveillance protocol as outlined by your individual skilled oncologist. ■

Bradley Somer, MD

Q: *Treatment for invasive colon cancer.* I have a friend in his early 40s who has recently been diagnosed with invasive colon adenocarcinoma. He underwent a colectomy with tumor resection. The tumor had invaded bladder, but without penetration. Surgical margins were clear of tumor, but 3/31 mesenteric nodes were positive. What is his prognosis, what are the treatment options, and is radiation treatment recommended? What are the likely results of treatment?

Standard treatment for colon cancer with positive nodes is adjuvant chemotherapy for several months. Chemotherapy may consist of 5-fluorouracil (5-FU) combined with levamisole for 12 months or 5-FU combined with leucovorin for 6 months following surgery. The 5-year survival in patients with 1–4 positive nodes is approximately 60% and better than in those patients with more than 4 positive nodes.

In contrast to rectal cancer, the role of adjuvant radiation therapy for cancers that arise above the pelvic peritoneal reflection has not been well established. Due to the anatomical locations of these cancers, particularly where the colon is attached to a mesentery, wide local resections are feasible. The primary failure pattern following potentially curative surgery is abdominal rather than local. When the tumor invades adjacent organs, such as the bladder, the risk of local relapse increases.

> " Standard treatment for colon cancer with positive nodes is adjuvant chemotherapy for several months

Retrospective non-randomized studies of radiation therapy following curative surgery of colon cancer with or without chemotherapy have suggested a potential benefit to both locoregional control, and perhaps disease-free survival as well, over surgical resection alone. It has been found that radiation therapy in addition to surgery significantly improves local control and recurrence-free survival rates in patients with a perforation or fistula associated with their tumor (stage B3) and those with stage C3 cancer (stage B3 plus local lymph node spread). Concurrent administration of 5-FU with the radiation therapy appears to improve local control compared to surgery plus radiation therapy only (79% versus 67% for stage C3 cancer), but the difference is not statistically significant.

There are more than a dozen clinical trials sponsored by the National Cancer Institute, which can be found at cancernet.nci.nih.gov/prot/patsrch.shtml.

You should ask your friend to talk to his oncologists to explore the treatment options. ■

Li Liu, MD

There has been much attention in the popular press to an avenue of treatment that blocks the blood vessel formation that tumors need to grow and spread to other areas. This class of drugs is called angiogenesis inhibitors. There has been speculation for many years that angiogenesis inhibitors provide a fruitful strategy for treating cancer. The first drug of this type that has shown significant success and gained approval in the United States for the treatment of metastatic colorectal cancer is called bevacizumab (Avastin).

Bevacizumab is a monoclonal antibody that binds to and inhibits the activity of vascular endothelial growth factor (VEGF). Hence, it inhibits the interaction of VEGF with its receptor on endothelial cells (lining of blood vessel). This, in turn, inhibits the proliferation of endothelial cells and thus inhibits new blood vessel formation. In essence, then, it kills tumors by cutting off its own blood supply.

Bevacizumab is administered intravenously, dosed individually, according to the patient's body mass. The dose used is 5 mg/kg every 2 weeks. The total dosage is delivered over 90 minutes as an initial infusion. If the first dose is well tolerated, the second infusion can be administered over 60 minutes. If this is well tolerated as well, subsequent infusions can be given over 30 minutes. No premedication is needed prior to the administration of bevacizumab.

> There has been speculation for many years that angiogenesis inhibitors provide a fruitful strategy for treating cancer

It should be noted that the approval for bevacizumab is derived from two large, randomized clinical trials in which bevacizumab was combined with either IFL chemotherapy (irinotecan, 5-fluorouracil [5-FU], leucovorin) or 5-fluorouracil and leucovorin chemotherapy. Bevacizumab is not approved as a single agent.

Although bevacizumab is well tolerated in most patients, it does have some unique side effects. Minor nosebleeds are common and not of major concern, but there are reports of rare serious bleeding episodes. High blood pressure may be caused by this medication, and blood pressure should be monitored regularly. There is a slightly higher rate of congestive heart failure in patients taking this medication. Gastrointestinal perforation (the development of an abnormal break in the wall of the stomach, intestines, or colon) occurred very rarely in some patients treated with bevacizumab. These episodes often resulted in an abscess formation. This may be due to the impaired wound healing induced by bevacizumab. Therefore, it is recommended that bevacizumab not be given within at least 28 days following major surgery. In addition, the surgical incision should be fully healed prior to initiation of bevacizumab. Although this is a severe complication, the risk is small. The typical presentation of wound breakdown and gastrointestinal perforation is abdominal pain (often severe) with associated constipation and/or vomiting. Therefore, any severe abdominal pain should be regarded as an emergency. Obviously, discontinuation of bevacizumab is warranted in these instances. ■

Bruce Giantonio, MD

Q: *Chemotherapy and follow-up after stage B2 colon cancer. I was diagnosed with stage II colon cancer in September 2000 at age 39. During a bowel resection 21 lymph nodes were removed (all negative). There was no apparent spread of tumor, but there was angiolymphatic invasion. The tumor was classified as stage B2. I am just completing six rounds of 5-fluorouracil (5-FU) and leucovorin. My concern is that 5-FU is an old drug and I've learned that it really doesn't offer much in terms of percentage of survival. Is there any other treatment available for stage B2 cancer, and what follow-up care would you recommend?*

The current recommendations are that patients receive 5-FU and leucovorin for this stage of colon cancer. We know that people with stage B2 colon cancer have a 75–80% chance of being cured with surgery alone. There is some controversy whether 5-FU chemotherapy benefits stage B2 patients, but some oncologists believe it does, and in younger patients it is reasonable to be aggressive in the overall treatment.

In terms of follow-up, a reasonable recommendation might be follow-up visits with an oncologist or surgeon every 3 months for 2–3 years, with blood work (including a serum carcinoembryonic antigen (CEA) level) performed at each visit, and thereafter annual follow-up visits. Many

66
follow-up visits with an oncologist or surgeon every 3 months for 2–3 years, with blood work

oncologists may also perform an annual chest x-ray, but there is some controversy regarding this. A colonoscopy may be performed 1 year after the surgery, and then annually or every 3 years depending on the findings of the postoperative examination. ■

James P Stevenson, MD

Chemotherapy for mucinous adenocarcinoma of the colon. What you could tell me about mucinous adenocarcinoma of the colon and a new treatment using a combination of CPT11, 5-fluorouracil, and leucovoran?

Mucinous adenocarcinoma is a term that describes the way this colon cancer looks under a microscope. We treat it the same way as any other colon cancer. The CPT11, 5-fluorouracil (5-FU), and leucovorin combination is now the standard first-line treatment for metastatic colon cancer. Each of these drugs has been found to be active against colon cancer. Multiple studies have shown that by combining these drugs better tumor response rates (about 50%) and longer survival of patients can be expected than when they are used alone.

The treatments are given once weekly for four consecutive weeks followed by a 2-week break period with no treatment. These 6-week cycles can be repeated if there are signs of improvement. Randomized trials are looking at adding newer drugs to this combination, such as anti-VEGF and celecoxib. The trials may be available in your area, and you could ask your oncologist if you may be eligible for any of these studies. ■

James P Stevenson, MD

> **"** by combining these drugs better tumor response rates (about 50%) and longer survival of patients can be expected than when they are used alone

Q: Treatment options after failed chemotherapy.
What can be done for a 60-year-old male with stage IV
colon cancer with metastases to the liver and extra-hepatic
disease? Multiple regimens of chemotherapy have failed.
The patient currently has an elevated bilirubin and is
receiving 5-fluorouracil (5-FU) via a portable intravenous
pump.

This is a difficult situation. Given an elevated bilirubin level, it may be advisable to continue with the 5-FU for as long as is possible. In addition, it may be helpful to consult with the treating oncologist to determine if the obstructed areas in the bile ducts can be drained in any way. Many times this is done by an interventional radiologist. If the 5-FU stops working, it may be advisable to explore available phase I clinical trials. ■

James P Stevenson, MD

> consult with the treating oncologist
> to determine if the obstructed areas in
> the bile ducts can be drained in any
> way

Diet and chemotherapy. My mother-in-law is undergoing chemotherapy. Her taste for food and her appetite are gone. She is becoming very weak. What can we do to boost her appetite or to infuse the small portions of food she is eating to modify the nutritional value?

When a person is struggling with a poor appetite, eating small frequent meals may help them meet their nutritional needs. The easiest plan is to eat smaller portions at meal times, but then include a snack or nutritious drink in between. Suggestions for snacks include peanut butter and crackers, deviled eggs, pudding, yogurt, or a breakfast bar. Commercial supplement drinks such as Ensure® or Boost® can be used, and Carnation Instant Breakfast®, Ovaltine®, and hot cocoa are good sources of calories and protein. Try to include some protein in every mini-meal.

Calculate your mother-in-law's calorie needs by using the following formula (1 pound = 0.45 kg):

calorie goal = 10 calories × weight in pounds

This will give you a goal to work towards. Keep a food diary in which you write down what is eaten, the time, and the number of calories consumed. Reviewing the log will help you identify ways to increase her intake.

Remember that fluid is also very important and often forgotten. Symptoms caused by dehydration, such as fatigue, dizziness, and nausea, are often blamed on other problems. The average person needs 64 fl oz

> " eat smaller portions at meal times, but then include a snack or nutritious drink in between

(1.9 liters) of fluids a day. By encouraging your mother-in-law to drink fluids that contain calories, such as juice and sodas, you can achieve two goals at the same time.

The cancer center where your mother receives her chemotherapy should have a registered dietitian available to meet with you and develop an individualized diet plan for your mother-in-law. ■

Katrina VB Claghorn, MS, RD

The answer to this question is dependent on the stage of the cancer In stage II or III colon cancer, chemotherapy after surgery (also called adjuvant therapy) is given in an effort to prevent the cancer from returning (or recurring). Forty percent of patients that have their entire tumor removed surgically will ultimately develop a recurrence. Chemotherapy can significantly decrease the chance of the cancer returning.

In stage IV colon cancer, chemotherapy after surgery is given to extend life or improve quality of life by alleviating symptoms caused by the tumor. Chemotherapy in these cases is not considered to cure a patient. Despite the fact that the primary tumor (the tumor in the colon) may have been removed by the surgeon, it has been determined that the cancer has spread to other organs. In a very small number of cases, it may be possible to surgically remove tumors in the liver or lung, improving the patient's chance for survival. Advances in chemotherapy have allowed patients with stage IV colon cancer to survive longer than ever before. ■

Carolyn Coyle, MSN, RN, AOCN

" dependent on the stage of the cancer

Treatment with 5-fluorouracil (5-FU) chemotherapy. Is it best to have 5-FU intravenously, by continuous infusion, or in pill form?

This is a difficult question to answer, as the treatment should fit the patient's particular case. For example, an elderly patient may not tolerate certain regimens as well as a younger, healthier patient, or a patient may not have responded to one form of 5-FU, but could respond to another form.

That being said, the oldest, and most tested way to receive 5-FU is by intravenous infusion, usually given over 2 hours. Studies have been testing this form of 5-FU since the 1950s. This is the method most often used in the treatment of stage II and III colon cancers after surgery, and in combination with other medications for stage IV cancer.

Several studies in the treatment of stage IV colon cancer have utilized continuous infusion 5-FU. These studies have reported decreased side-effects, and some have reported increased response rates with a small benefit in survival time. This method of giving 5-FU may be used in conjunction with 5-FU by shorter infusion, other chemotherapies, or radiation.

Oral 5-FU is a relatively new treatment available for the treatment of colon cancers. In one study more responses to treatment were found when 5-FU was given orally than when it was given by infusion, but the time until the cancer returned or progressed was equal with both medication routes. Because it works differently than the intravenous form, oral 5-FU may be an option for patients who no longer respond to the intravenous form. ■

Carolyn Coyle, MSN, RN, AOCN

66
the treatment should fit the patient's particular case

Chemotherapy and side-effects. What are the side-effects of the most common chemotherapy drugs used for colorectal cancer?

Chemotherapy kills cells that divide rapidly. Unfortunately, this includes both good cells (hair follicles, mucosa of the mouth and the gastrointestinal tract, red and white blood cells, etc.) and bad cells (tumor). Every chemotherapy has slightly different side-effects, which vary from patient to patient. The following paragraphs describe the most common side-effects for each medication and some ways to manage them.

FLUOROURACIL (5-FU)

Diarrhea. This can often be managed with loperamide (Imodium) or lomotil (antidiarrheal medications). A doctor or nurse can give you instructions on how to take these medications, as this will often differ from the instructions on the box. Patients with diarrhea should drink plenty of non-alcoholic fluids to prevent dehydration. Diarrhea can be very serious and require a reduction in the dose of chemotherapy, so be sure to let your physician know if you have it.

Mouth sores. Patients should get into the habit of rinsing their mouth with sterile water (or normal saline) or a mouth rinse that does not contain alcohol. If you do get mouth sores, your doctor or nurse can suggest a numbing mouth rinse (Magic Mouthwash®, Xylocaine®, or Hurricane®) to ease any discomfort. Popsicles or soft, cold foods may

66
Every chemotherapy has slightly different side-effects, which vary from patient to patient

feel soothing to a sore mouth. Avoid spicy or hot foods, as these might irritate the mouth.

Eye problems. Patients may notice gritty or watery eyes. Lubricating drops, such as normal saline, can help with gritty, irritated eyes. This is temporary and should go away after treatments are stopped.

Lowering of blood counts. Effects on blood counts vary depending on the dose and schedule of chemotherapy. Your doctor or nurse can tell you what to expect in your particular case. A low hemoglobin (the cell that carries oxygen) count is called 'anemia', and can make you feel tired or, when more severe, short of breath. A low platelet count leads to easy bruising and bleeding, and a low white blood cell count puts a patient at higher risk for infection. While receiving chemotherapy you should notify your doctor or nurse if you have a temperature above 100.5°C or experience easy bruising or bleeding.

Changes to nails and skin. Nails can become dark, brittle, and chipped. These changes will grow out when treatment is stopped. Skin may also darken, particularly around the veins where the chemotherapy is given. These changes are also temporary. In addition, a patient's skin is more sensitive to sunlight, and may burn easier than usual, so be sure to use sunscreen and avoid sun exposure.

Less common side-effects include the following.

Nausea and vomiting. There are several types of medications available to treat nausea and vomiting. You should let your doctor know if you have nausea or vomiting so they can give you medications to prevent this. You should stick to a bland diet (chicken broth, toast, rice) when feeling sick and be sure to drink plenty of fluids.

Hair loss. This is not too common with 5-FU treatment, but you may notice thinning of your hair. This usually starts about 3–4 weeks after treatment has begun. Hair will grow back after therapy is finished.

Soreness or redness of the palms. Also called palmar–plantar syndrome, or hand and foot syndrome. This is a reddening and peeling of the soles of the feet and the palms of the hands, which can become severe if treatment is not stopped to allow heeling. It is most commonly seen with the continuous infusion or oral forms of 5-FU (capecitabine (Xeloda)).

Reaction during infusion. Some patients may experience sweating, watery eyes, abdominal cramping, and diarrhea during the infusion. If this happens, a medication called atropine is given to stop or prevent the symptoms.

Diarrhea. The most common side-effect of this medication is diarrhea. It typically starts a few days after treatment, and can be severe. Your doctor or nurse should provide you with special instructions on how to take loperamide (Imodium), as this will be different from the instructions on the box. It is very important to let your doctor know how severe the diarrhea is (usually by the number of bowel movements per day). This may require your chemotherapy dose to be decreased. It is also important to drink a lot of fluids when you have diarrhea.

Nausea and vomiting. There are several types of medication available to treat nausea and vomiting. You should let your doctor know if you have nausea or vomiting so they can give you medications to prevent this. You should stick to a bland diet (chicken broth, toast, rice) when feeling sick and be sure to drink plenty of fluids.

Lowering of blood counts. Blood counts reach their lowest point 7–10 days after treatment and return to normal about 21 days after treatment. Effects on blood counts vary depending on the dose and schedule of chemotherapy. Your doctor or nurse can tell you what to expect in your particular case. A low hemoglobin (the cell that carries oxygen) count is called 'anemia' and can make you feel tired or, when more severe, short of breath. A low platelet count leads to easy bruising and bleeding, and a low white blood cell count puts a patient at higher risk for infection. While receiving chemotherapy you should notify your doctor or nurse if you have a temperature above 100.5°C or experience easy bruising or bleeding.

Hair loss. This usually begins 3–4 weeks after starting treatment, but can begin earlier. You may lose all your hair, including eyebrows, eyelashes, and other body hair. Hair will grow back after treatments are completed, although it may be different in color or texture than before treatment. In the meantime you may choose to wear a wig, hat, or scarf. If you choose to wear a wig it is a good idea to get one before you lose your hair, so you can match it to your natural color. In the cold weather it is helpful to wear a hat to keep warm.

Less common side-effects are as follows.

Mouth sores. Patients should get into the habit of rinsing their mouth with sterile water (normal saline) or a mouth rinse that does not contain alcohol. If you do get mouth sores, your doctor or nurse can suggest a numbing mouth rinse (Magic Mouthwash, Xylocaine, and Hurricane) to alleviate any discomfort. Popsicles or soft, cold foods may feel soothing to a sore mouth. Avoid spicy or hot foods, as these might irritate the mouth.

Skin rash. CPT-11 (Irinotecan) can cause an itchy rash. If this occurs, let your doctor know. A medication can be prescribed to help with the itching.

OXALIPLATIN

Numbness or tingling. Patients often report a numb or tingling feeling in their hands, feet, or throat. Often this is brought on by cold (e.g. drinking a cold drink or touching a cold steering wheel). It may not occur until after several treatments, and may get worse over the course of treatments, but should return to normal once treatments are stopped. To help with cold-related feelings you should avoid cold beverages, wear gloves in the cold weather, and bundle up when going outside in cold weather or into air-conditioned buildings.

Lowering of blood counts. The blood counts reach their lowest point 7–10 days after treatment, then increase slowly, returning to normal 21–28 days after treatment. Your doctor or nurse can tell you what to expect in your particular case. A low hemoglobin (the cell that carries oxygen) count is called 'anemia' and can make you feel tired or, when more severe, short of breath. A low platelet count leads to easy bruising and bleeding, and a low white blood cell count puts a patient at higher risk for infection. While receiving chemotherapy you should notify your doctor or nurse if you have a temperature above 100.5°C or experience easy bruising or bleeding.

Nausea and vomiting. There are several types of medication available to treat nausea and vomiting. You should let your doctor know if you have nausea or vomiting so they can give you medications to prevent this. You should stick to a bland diet (chicken broth, toast, rice) when feeling sick and be sure to drink plenty of fluids.

Diarrhea. This can often be managed with loperamide (Imodium) or lomotil (antidiarrheal medications). A doctor or nurse can give you instructions on how to take these. Patients with diarrhea should drink plenty of non-alcoholic fluids to prevent dehydration. Diarrhea can be very serious and require a reduction in the dose of chemotherapy, so be sure to let your physician know if you have it.

Less common side-effects are as follows.

Allergic reactions. A few patients may have an allergic reaction to this medication. This may present during the infusion as hives and itching, shivering, a high temperature, redness of the face, shortness of breath, or anxiety. Let your nurse know immediately if you experience these symptoms. A medication can be given to reverse the reaction and, for future doses, medication can be taken prior to the chemotherapy to prevent this reaction.

Mouth sores. Patients should get into the habit of rinsing their mouth with sterile water (normal saline) or a mouth rinse that does not contain alcohol. If you do get mouth sores, your doctor or nurse can suggest a numbing mouth rinse (Magic Mouthwash®, Xylocaine®, and Hurricane®) to help alleviate any discomfort. Popsicles or soft, cold foods may feel soothing to a sore mouth. Avoid spicy or hot foods, as these might irritate the mouth. ■

Carolyn Coyle, MSN, RN, AOCN

Chemotherapy and Crohn's disease. How might chemotherapy affect Crohn's disease? Do you have any special dietary recommendations for a patient with Crohn's?

There has been little research on how chemotherapy for cancer affects Crohn's disease. For a patient with a history of Crohn's disease, we would recommend the same dietary management of gastrointestinal side-effects as for any other patient receiving chemotherapy.

If any diarrhea develops, the recommendations would be a soft, lactose-free diet and adequate fluid intake (48–64 fl oz/day (1.4–1.9 liter/day)) to prevent dehydration. The side-effects will also depend on the particular drugs used to treat the cancer. Some drugs have more gastrointestinal side-effects than others. If the patient's intake and weight are being affected, I would recommend a consultation with a dietitian to evaluate the situation fully. ■

Ellen Sweeney-Cordes, MS, RD

> 66
> the same dietary management of
> gastrointestinal side-effects as for any
> other patient receiving chemotherapy

Q: *Oxaliplatin (Eloxatin) and 5-FU. I am 65 years old and have been diagnosed with recurrent colon cancer in the liver. I previously was treated with surgery followed by 5-FU chemotherapy 3 years ago when I had 4 lymph nodes with cancer. My doctors are now recommending a treatment course with oxaliplatin and 5-FU. Is this standard treatment? What side-effects may I experience?*

Although experiencing a recurrence of colon cancer can be difficult, there are new options to manage recurrent colon cancer that were not available when you were initially diagnosed with cancer 3 years ago. Oxaliplatin (Eloxatin) was approved by the US FDA for treatment of metastatic colorectal cancer in August of 2002. Oxaliplatin works by interfering with the replication of cancer cells. Oxaliplatin appears to enhance the effects of 5-FU when they are given together. This combination is frequently referred to as FOLFOX. This has become one of the available standard regimens for metastatic colorectal cancer.

Side-effects, although slightly more numerous than those seen with 5-FU alone, are very tolerable. One of the unique side-effects of oxaliplatin is numbness or tingling in the hands, feet, and/or throat when exposed to cold. Avoid exposure to the cold, especially on the day of treatment. Wear gloves and socks to protect hands and feet. Cold food and drink can cause a feeling of numbness and tingling in the throat, so avoid these on treatment days. This side effect can last for a day or two, but then should improve. Notify your healthcare provider if these symptoms persist. Other side-effects may include nausea, vomiting, diarrhea, and

> " there are new options to manage recurrent colon cancer that were not available when you were initially diagnosed

a decrease in blood counts. These side-effects are generally mild and manageable with your oncologist but may require a reduction in the next dose of oxaliplatin.

In very select patients, surgery may be performed after chemotherapy to remove an isolated metastasis in the liver or metastases involving a single lobe of the liver. This must be individualized and discussed with your oncology team. ■

Daniel G. Haller, MD

Q: *Combination of oxaliplatin (Eloxatin), 5-FU, and leucovorin. I recently had surgery for colon cancer. The surgeon told me that everything was taken out, but the tumor did extend through the muscle wall and there was 1 lymph node out of 15 with cancer. I did meet with a medical oncologist who told me that I need chemotherapy. I am starting treatment next week with 5-FU and oxaliplatin. Does this sound like a reasonable recommendation?*

For patients in your situation, chemotherapy is considered standard treatment. Based on your description, this was a stage III tumor that was completely removed at surgery. However, based on numerous studies, chemotherapy is indicated due to a high risk of microscopic residual cancer, and 5-FU with leucovorin has been a standard therapy for a number of years. There was a very large, randomized study published in the *New England Journal of Medicine* in June 2004 that randomized patients after surgery between standard 5-FU and leucovorin chemotherapy versus 5-FU and leucovorin with oxaliplatin (Eloxatin). The patients with stage III disease who received the oxaliplatin regimen had a significant improvement in disease-free survival at 4-year follow-up. There was an 8.7% absolute improvement in disease-free survival and a 25% relative risk reduction in recurrence. Based on this study, the combination of

66

The combination of oxaliplatin (Eloxatin), 5-FU, and leucovorin is now considered a standard of care for stage III colon cancer oxaliplatin, 5-FU, and leucovorin is now considered a standard of care for stage III colon cancer after surgical resection. ■

Daniel G. Haller, MD

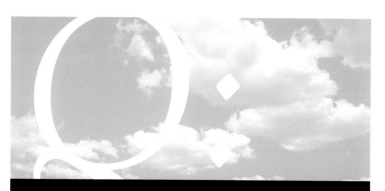

Treatment – Radiation Therapy

Q: *Risks of radiation therapy for a lupus patient.*
Can a patient with lupus and rectal cancer have a
radiation therapy treatment? If so, what will be the risks?

The answer is yes, although there is a high risk of excessive skin reaction and subcutaneous fibrosis (skin thickening) and a smaller chance of pelvic fibrosis (scarring). It is recommended that the radiation oncologist use the highest available energy (15–18 MV to minimize skin dose).

The rheumatologist should do as much as possible to quiet the lupus down before starting radiation. Antimetabolite chemotherapy (methotrexate and azothioprine) may be given to patients with lupus with salutary results. 5-Fluorouracil (5-FU) is also an antimetabolite that is commonly given. It is unclear if it reduces the fibrosis that can be associated with radiation treatment in this population. ■

Richard Whittington, MD

66

there is a high risk of excessive skin
reaction and subcutaneous fibrosis
(skin thickening) and a smaller chance
of pelvic fibrosis (scarring)

Side-effects of radiation to the rectum. What are the side-effects of radiation treatment to the rectum?

This is a question with two answers, since there are early and late side-effects that can occur. The early effects of radiation to the rectum usually are minimal. The initial response is irritation. The rectum is a mucous membrane and, like any mucous membrane, when irritated it makes extra mucous. Think about pollen or dust irritating your nose. People find their bowel movements are softer, 'slippery', and more frequent. Some people will even leak a little brown mucous when they pass gas.

Other effects include bladder irritation with urinary frequency, urgency, and nocturia (urination at night). The skin around the area may get a sunburn and possibly peel; there is irritation of the vagina in women, with dryness and adhesions in the vagina. Many women will go through menopause. There is a small risk of impotence in men.

Late effects of radiation for rectal cancer, which is usually done in conjunction with surgery, may rarely cause ulcers or stricture (<5% risk). With higher doses there is a risk of an ulcer. This usually occurs 12–36 months after radiation in a patch of scar tissue and is frequently caused by a scratch or other break in the mucous membrane. This allows a local infection to start and the tissue in the scar will die, producing an ulcer. This is because the blood supply to the surface is reduced and the body has trouble fighting the infection, which allows the ulcer to get bigger. The infection causes swelling and the blood supply is further reduced. This is treated classically by applying a steroid enema or

" there are early and late side-effects that can occur

suppository to reduce the inflammation and thus to increase the blood supply to facilitate healing. It also will interfere with the immune response to the infection. Recently, gastroenterologists have been looking at a new technique where they laser the surface to stop the bleeding. Some physicians use the drug carafate (sucralfate), which was developed to treat stomach ulcers. It is sort of like spackling compound for the intestine and will stick to the inflamed areas. It promotes growth of the mucosa and is antibacterial. This seems to work pretty well in most patients. The final late effect due to scarring is that, because the fibrosis contracts as it matures, it is possible to get a stricture. Surgery may rarely be required to deal with this complication. ■

Richard Whittington, MD

Q:

Side-effects of radiation to the colon. I had radiation therapy ending in December 2000 after a tumor was removed from my colon. Since then I have experienced irregular bowel movements, cramps, constipation, and diarrhea. There is also a mucus discharge. My oncologists all agree that the problems are related to the radiation, but do not give much other information. What could this be?

Your symptoms may be the result of irradiation, but it is uncommon for them to last this long. The doctors first need to rule out other causes, including short bowel or short colon syndrome after surgery, infections with *Helicobacter*, *Clostridium difficile*, *Shigella*, or the like, hypersecretory state after surgery, lactose intolerance after surgery or chemotherapy, pancreatic insufficiency, partial small bowel obstruction due to surgical adhesions, and colorrhetic diarrhea due to bile salts. Less frequent causes are sprue-like syndromes. When all these possibilities have been ruled out it is possible to think about radiation as a cause if the dose was high enough and the field was large enough to include a lot of the small bowel. This is very rare. There is a tendency among other physicians to assume every unpleasant thing that happens after a person has undergone radiation therapy is due to a radiation injury. This is rare, and is usually seen only after whole abdominal doses greater than 22 Gy. Work-up could consist of an upper gastrointestinal with small bowel follow through, endoscopy (upper or lower), and possibly small bowel aspirate or biopsy. ■

Richard Whittington, MD

> **"** The doctors first need to rule out other causes

Q: *Neurologic deficits after radiation for colorectal cancer. My mother underwent surgery for colorectal cancer 3 years ago. She was treated with chemotherapy as well as radiation. She did fine until one of her last radiation treatments. At that point, she started having pain in her hips, back, and legs. She was diagnosed with a ruptured disk and had additional surgery. The back pain subsided to a degree, but her other symptoms have continued. Can radiation cause this reaction?*

It is not possible to say for certain whether the problem is related to the radiation. The time course is incorrect, as this complication usually occurs 6–24 months after radiation, although with higher doses it is possible to occur earlier. Many of her neurological deficits are probably arising from fibrosis in the region of the ruptured disk. This can be caused by surgery and by the ruptured disk, as well as by any bleeding that may have occurred in the region. Radiation would make this fibrosis denser and may exacerbate the problem, but would be unlikely to be the cause of it. ▪

Richard Whittington, MD

" this complication usually occurs 6–24 months after radiation

Q: *Radiation prior to surgery for rectal cancer. I have recently been diagnosed with rectal cancer. I was told that chemotherapy and radiation are required before surgery. The mass is approximately 10 cm. Frankly, I would rather have surgery first. What are your thoughts on this matter?*

Radiation given before the surgery is better tolerated because the tissues that are going to be removed with surgery are still in place and they push the normal tissues out of the way. This way there is less radiation to normal tissue, which is good. If radiation is given after surgery, the small intestine will fall into the area where the tumor was located and it may get unnecessary radiation. An additional problem is that some people may have scarring of the bowels and there is an increased risk of intestinal blockage when radiation is delivered after the surgery.

Another benefit of preoperative treatment is that radiation may be able to change the surgical approach in those patients who would normally require a permanent colostomy. If the tumor can be shrunk with radiation and chemotherapy, it may be possible to avoid a permanent colostomy. Some patients may still need a temporary colostomy after preoperative chemotherapy and radiation because it slows the healing and is usually closed 4–6 months after surgery.

The downside to treating all patients with preoperative radiation is that some will be treated with radiation unnecessarily. Because the tests used to evaluate the extent of the tumor (computed tomography (CT),

> " radiation may be able to change the surgical approach in those patients that would normally require a permanent colostomy

ultrasound, magnetic resonance imaging (MRI), etc.) are not perfect, some patients who probably could have been treated with surgery only will receive radiation. This is the major reason why postoperative treatment may be favored, unless it is clear from the physical examination and radiology tests that the patient will require radiation therapy even after surgery.

There are a large number of institutions that do it each way, and it would be best to talk to a doctor who does postoperative treatment routinely and ask them what their opinion is and why.

As a general rule, patients with a tumor that does not penetrate the bowel wall and where there is no involvement of lymph nodes do not need any treatment other than surgery. If the preoperative testing suggests the tumor has broken through the bowel wall or is stuck to other tissues, or there are enlarged lymph nodes, then that patient may need radiation and chemotherapy. The latter group is routinely treated preoperatively with chemotherapy and radiation before surgery, followed by additional chemotherapy after surgery. The former group may be recommended to have surgery and, if the physicians are unpleasantly surprised by the extent of the tumor, these patients may be given chemotherapy and radiation after surgery. ■

Richard Whittington, MD

Cancer of the colon and rectum are actually the same tumor in different locations. When the surgeon takes out the tumor, treatment depends on the margin of safety of the removal. The easiest way to think about this is as if the colon and rectum are a length of pipe. Tumors that break through the wall are like a leak in the pipe that may contaminate the surrounding soil and tumor cells in lymphatic fluid and lymph nodes are like ground water contamination. When the colon is inside the peritoneal cavity of the abdomen it moves about as if it is on a very long tether drawing its blood supply through the long thin sheet of the mesentery. This is as if the pipe is elevated on a platform. There is not any nearby soil to become contaminated. The surgeon gets a wide margin of safety around the tumor like the pipeline maintenance crew can remove the defective segment of pipe and the platform to prevent contamination of the surrounding soil. However, it is possible for the tumor to spread to lymph glands, as the leak in the pipe may contaminate ground water. In the last 6 inches of its course the colon becomes the rectum, which simply means it leaves the peritoneal cavity. Here it may lie on the bladder, the uterus, the prostate, or the sacrum (tail bone), which cannot be safely removed. It is as if the pipe were lying on a rock field that is too big and extensive to remove. Here there is a risk of contamination of the surrounding soil as well as the ground water. Since there are much higher concentrations of contaminants on the soil than in the ground water, they are managed differently.

66

radiation is more effective at dealing with a higher concentration of tumor cells, but can only be used to treat a defined area

Booms and sponges are used to mop up as much of the contamination as possible, because the concentrations are so high. Detergents and other chemicals are used to treat the remaining contamination and the ground water. Similarly, radiation is more effective at dealing with a higher concentration of tumor cells, but can only be used to treat a defined area, not the whole body, while chemotherapy can treat isolated cells and does treat the whole body. We have also found that chemotherapy will make tumor cells more sensitive to the effects of radiation, without having anywhere near the same effect on normal cells. This is why chemotherapy and radiation are used together. In several trials comparison has been made between surgery alone, surgery + chemotherapy, surgery + radiation therapy, and surgery + radiation therapy + chemotherapy. In general, it was found that chemotherapy delayed the regrowth of tumor in the tissues around the original tumor but the overall risk did not appreciably change. Thus patients lived longer but there was only a small increase in the cure rate. Radiation sharply reduced the risk of any regrowth of the tumor in the surrounding tissues but did not have much effect on the risk of spread elsewhere in the body and did not increase the cure rate at all. The combination of radiation and chemotherapy effectively treated both problems and did increase the cure rate. The questions now are which chemotherapy and what tumors need radiation? In general, radiation is not given for tumors of the colon inside the peritoneal cavity, unless the tumor is stuck to something or growing into another organ (T4 tumor). Chemotherapy is used when the lymph nodes are involved and when radiation is given for a T4 tumor. In the last 6 inches of the colon, the rectum, chemotherapy and radiation are given when a tumor has broken through the wall of the rectum, even if it is not stuck to anything, and when the lymph nodes are involved. ▪

Richard Whittington, MD

Timing of surgery after radiation. How long do I need to wait after surgery before radiation?

In general, you wait until the surgeon says that healing is adequate for you to receive radiation. This is generally 3–6 weeks after surgery, but may be longer if there are postoperative problems that delay healing. Since chemotherapy is given with the radiation, the two may start together or the radiation can be delayed for 2 or possibly 4 months after chemotherapy started without losing any of its effectiveness. ■

Richard Whittington, MD

66
This is generally 3–6 weeks after surgery

Radiation to improve surgical removal of colon cancer. My doctor said I could have radiation before surgery to 'shrink the tumor' and avoid a colostomy. Can you tell me more about this?

When surgeons operate they go above and below the tumor by a couple of inches to be certain they get an adequate margin around the tumor. If the lower margin is too close to the anus (the opening of the rectum to the outside) then it is necessary to put in a colostomy. If the radiation and chemotherapy shrink the tumor and it is not as close to the anus, it may be possible to avoid a colostomy. When radiation is used preoperatively, less of a margin of safety is needed around the tumor and the patient may be spared a colostomy. The preoperative treatment is similar to the radiation and chemotherapy that is recommended in the postoperative setting. However, the patient generally receives additional chemotherapy after the surgery has been completed. Sometimes surgeons will put in a temporary colostomy to allow the bowel that has been connected time to heal. This colostomy can be removed after adequate healing time (usually a few months). ■

Richard Whittington, MD

66
When radiation is used preoperatively less of a margin of safety is needed around the tumor

Chemotherapy blocks many of the repair activities of tumor cells without having the same effect on normal cells. This increases the sensitivity of tumor cells to the effects of radiation. There have been numerous clinical studies that show patients do much better when chemotherapy and radiation therapy are given concurrently. ■

Richard Whittington, MD

> **"** patients do much better when chemotherapy and radiation therapy are given concurrently

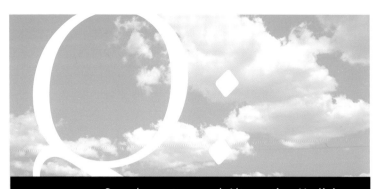

Complementary and Alternative Medicine

These terms are often used without a good understanding of the definitions. With the increased popularity of unconventional medical treatments, these terms are being used more and more. Here is a guide to help with the confusing jargon.

Conventional cancer therapies consist of those forms of cancer treatment that are widely practiced and have been proven beneficial in clinical research trials. These may include surgery, chemotherapy, radiation therapy, and/or hormonal therapy. These treatments are used in mainstream cancer centers throughout the world.

Unconventional cancer therapies are any approaches to the diagnosis, treatment, and care of the cancer patient that fall outside conventional cancer treatments. Many different categories of unconventional therapies have been described, including psychological techniques, specialized diets, herbal therapies, spiritual healers, traditional cultural techniques, and pharmacological treatments. Unconventional treatments have not been proven to cure cancer in scientific research trials. Some treatments have been shown to be beneficial in helping patients with the side-effects of their conventional medical treatments. Unconventional medical therapies fall into two broad categories: complementary and alternative.

Complementary cancer treatments are those unconventional cancer therapies used in conjunction with conventional medical treatments

> " Complementary cancer treatments are those unconventional cancer therapies used in conjunction with conventional medical treatments

(e.g. acupuncture and guided imagery used for nausea caused by chemotherapy).

Alternative cancer treatments are those unconventional cancer therapies that are used instead of conventional medical therapies. Always discuss any unconventional medical treatments that you are considering with your physician. Although these can be helpful, many can interact with your body and make it difficult for you to complete your conventional medical treatments that have been proven to cure cancer. ■

James M Metz, MD

> " Alternative cancer treatments are those unconventional cancer therapies that are used instead of conventional medical therapies

Hoax treatments. I see lots of things publicized on the Internet but I do not know what is real and what is a scam. How do I avoid the hoaxes that are promoted as new treatments for cancer by some people?

Unconventional medical treatments for cancer are gaining increasing exposure to the public though television, the Internet, and magazines. Some unconventional therapies may one day prove to help cancer patients. These therapies are generally classified as 'alternative' or 'unconventional' because they have not been proven to benefit cancer patients in controlled clinical trials. It is a challenge to differentiate those techniques that offer promise from those that are hoaxes.

Many individuals claim that natural products are better for combating cancer than are conventional treatments such as chemotherapy, radiation therapy, and surgery. However, just because something is natural does not mean it is effective and safe. Poison ivy is natural, but most patients would not go and rub it intentionally all over their body. It is true that many of the therapies used today were discovered in nature, but these have been isolated, standardized, and purified. They have also been rigorously tested in controlled clinical trials to establish the effectiveness of the agent and its side-effect profile.

Cancer patients are prime targets for unscrupulous individuals who attempt to gain financially from the misfortunes of others. Always remember, if a treatment sounds too good to be true, it may be a hoax. Here are some classic signs of a hoax that should place the cancer patient on the alert:

66
Always tell your doctor if you are considering any such treatment

- The treatment is a 'secret' that only specific individuals can provide.

- Patients are told not to use conventional medical treatment.

- The treatment promises a cure for almost all cancers or medical conditions.

- The treatment is only promoted in the mass media such as the Internet, talk shows, and books, instead of reputable scientific journals.

- The promoters claim they are persecuted by the medical establishment.

- Advertisements for the treatment claim to 'cleanse the body of poisons and toxins'.

- The treatment will help the patient by 'strengthening the immune system'.

- Testimonials and case reports are used to promote a specific treatment or product.

- Catch phrases such as 'non-toxic', 'no side-effects', and 'painless' are used.

- The promoters attack the medical community.

If you are considering an alternative or complementary treatment be cautious and aware of any of the above claims. Always tell your doctor if you are considering any such treatment. Certain treatments may be helpful, but others may interfere with your traditional treatments.

James M Metz, MD

A number of complementary medical techniques are gaining increased acceptance within the medical community. Some of the most accepted complementary techniques include the mind–body therapies. These include, to name just a few, meditation, biofeedback, guided imagery, music therapy, art therapy, prayer, and hypnosis. These techniques may help the patient deal with anxiety, stress, and other subjective symptoms related to the diagnosis and treatment of cancer.

Meditation is a good technique to help with stress reduction. It is an easy technique to learn and can be done without the help of a therapist. It can be practiced in a variety of places, including work, home, and in hospital. Meditation originated in the Eastern religions and was used for calming and focusing the mind. There are many ways to practice meditation, and each individual develops their own style and preferences. Most recommend performing meditation once or twice a day for 10–20 minutes to reap the full benefits. There are many good books available to those interested in learning meditation. Browse through your local bookstore at the selections. Meditation is a wonderful complementary medical technique that is safe, relaxing and, best of all, free!

Guided imagery is a technique that relies heavily on the power of suggestion to create relaxing mental images for the participants. It is particularly useful for relieving stress and relaxing the cancer patient. It is not a treatment for cancer, but some patients find it helps them cope

" These techniques may help the patient deal with anxiety, stress, and other subjective symptoms related to the diagnosis and treatment of cancer more effectively with the diagnosis and side-effects of treatments. The therapist will instruct the participants to visualize a specific image. The initial goal of guided imagery is total relaxation. Patients learn breathing exercises to help them attain an 'inner calm'. Patients then try to modify their anxiety or pain by imagining a pleasurable scene or situation. Many patients utilize guided imagery audiotapes, which provide instruction on meditation exercises, guided relaxation, and visualization techniques. Some patients use these tapes while they are receiving their chemotherapy, radiation therapy, or traveling to their treatments.

Biofeedback manipulates the body's physiologic responses that are normally controlled by the autonomic nervous system. A biofeedback therapist can teach a patient how to control many of the body's involuntary functions. Some patients learn to control their heart rate, blood pressure, muscle tension, and emotions. The therapist places monitoring electrodes on the body or scalp and connects them to a computer or polygraph. The latter emits a noise or signal indicating the intensity or level of the process to be controlled and the patient is then instructed to concentrate on trying to influence to signal. Specific mental exercises are performed under the direction of the therapist. The patient may eventually learn which mental exercises change the signals. After a number of sessions (usually 8–10) the patient may be able to affect certain autonomic processes. Biofeedback is a technique that can be useful in a wide variety of conditions, but it is not used to cure cancer. The greatest benefit from biofeedback for the cancer patient is relaxation and reduction of stress. This can undoubtedly improve the quality of life for those who are successful. Biofeedback is non-invasive, inexpensive, and safe. ■

James M Metz, MD

Q: *Chemotherapy and vitamins.* *I administer chemotherapy and have recently heard of a new study that shows vitamin therapy in cancer patients receiving chemotherapy to be non-therapeutic. Some of my patients tell me that the study states that vitamins help enhance cancer growth and cell resistance to chemotherapy. Do you know where I can get a copy of this study?*

There are actually several studies that show potential interactions between antioxidant vitamin supplementation (e.g. vitamins C, E, and A) and cancer treatments, both radiation and chemotherapy. The theory is that, since antioxidants protect the body's cells from oxidation or damage, taking excess amounts of them may also protect the cancerous cells from oxidative cancer treatments, therefore decreasing the effectiveness of the treatments. Since research is not yet conclusive in this area, it is usually recommended that patients avoid extra antioxidant supplements throughout treatment. A standard multivitamin that provides 100% of the recommended daily intake for vitamins and minerals is okay. The following are references to some studies that have been reported in respectable journals:

1. Hamilton KK 2001 Antioxidant supplements during cancer treatments: where do we stand? Clinical Journal of Oncology Nursing 5(4):181–182

2. Labriola D, Livingston R 1999 Possible interactions between dietary antioxidants and chemotherapy. Oncology 13:1003–1011

" cancer cells consume large amounts of vitamin C, therefore possibly protecting them from radiation or chemotherapy

3. Lamson DW, Brignall MS 1999 Antioxidants in cancer therapy: their actions and interactions with oncologic therapies. Alternative Medicine Review 4:304–329

4. Agus DB, Vera JC, Golde DW 1999 Stromal cell oxidation: a mechanism by which tumors obtain vitamin C. Cancer Research 59(18):4555–4558

The last study listed was done specifically with vitamin C and cancer cells and showed that cancer cells consume large amounts of vitamin C, therefore possibly protecting them from radiation or chemotherapy. This may be the study that your patients referred to, although it is not that recent. In addition, some large studies have shown that some patients, particularly those with lung cancer, have significantly worse overall survival with antioxidant supplementation. ■

Ellen Sweeney-Cordes, MS, RD

Q: *Glutamine during chemotherapy. I am presently receiving chemotherapy for a recurrence of cancer. I developed mouth sores during my last treatment cycle. I have read that oral glutamine can decrease the severity and duration of stomatitis. Are there any reasons why I should not take oral glutamine during my next treatment cycle?*

There have been several good studies indicating a reduction in the degree of stomatitis associated with cancer treatments when oral glutamine supplementation is used. It does not always work, but maybe worth trying. Glutamine is considered to be safe and non-toxic, but do discuss this with your physician before using it. The best results seen in research studies are when oral glutamine 'swish and swallow' is started 2 weeks prior to treatment, and continued through treatment and for 2 weeks following treatment. The glutamine should be the pure L-glutamine form and not contain any antioxidants. Some preparations have antioxidants added, which may be contraindicated with your other treatment. The usual dose is 10 mg glutamine powder three times daily (for a total of 30 mg/day) mixed into your favorite beverage, swished around your mouth, and swallowed. ■

Ellen Sweeney-Cordes, MS, RD

66

Glutamine is considered to be safe and non-toxic, but do discuss this with your physician before using it

Most cancer centers counsel patients against taking antioxidants during chemotherapy and radiation therapy since there is the possibility that they may reduce the effectiveness of the treatments. The rationale is that antioxidants may somehow protect the tumor during cytoreductive therapy. Also, since people often think more is better and may take large amounts of many of the antioxidants it is important to warn people about the potential impact on their treatment. However, the key word is 'potential', since there are no studies to support the assumption. It is important to understand that the recommendation to avoid antioxidant nutrients only applies during active cancer treatment. These nutrients can be very beneficial before and after therapy. ∎

Katrina VB Claghorn, MS, RD

66 These nutrients can be very beneficial before and after therapy

Q: *Antioxidants and chemotherapy.* My wife is set to begin chemotherapy treatment. We are working with a nutritional advisor. We will be following his 10-step program, which advocates exercise, a low fat, high fiber diet, meditation, and vitamin and mineral supplements. He is advocating continuing to use the vitamins during chemotherapy because there is no study that shows a negative effect on the treatment, while there are many studies supporting the use of antioxidants. Should my wife continue on the vitamin regimen during chemotherapy or not?

Actually there are studies showing that some antioxidants can interfere with chemotherapy. There have also been some studies showing benefit from combining antioxidants and chemotherapy. However, the problem is that we are still trying to figure out which antioxidants and which chemotherapies can be combined. So far there is not enough information to substantiate either claim. Your wife's medical team will develop a treatment regimen based on sound science and they will always lean towards the side of caution. The regimens they use have been tested and the potential problems identified. The effect of using antioxidants with these treatments has not received the same scientific scrutiny, which is why there is hesitancy to combine them outside of clinical trials. If your wife is receiving radiation therapy, she should stop using antioxidants.

" we are still trying to figure out which antioxidants and which chemotherapies can be combined

Radiation therapy kills cancer cells by generating oxidants. If high doses of antioxidants are present, this could theoretically decrease the effectiveness of radiation treatments. ■

Katrina VB Claghorn, MS, RD

Q: *Grapeseed extract and chemotherapy.* *I am considering taking grapeseed during chemotherapy. Are there studies that show whether the antioxidants in grapeseed are beneficial in my situation?*

I am assuming you want to take grapeseed extract for its antioxidant effects, which may be beneficial in preventing cancer. However, there is potential that the antioxidant activity of grapeseed may interfere with chemotherapy and radiation therapies. These therapies produce oxidizing free radicals and their action could be limited by the presence of antioxidants, which as the name implies are antagonist to the oxidative process.

Studies assessing the affect of antioxidants on chemotherapy have been limited to test tube and animal studies, and the results have been conflicting. Part of the problem is that the different antioxidants vary in how they interact with the chemotherapeutic agents.

While antioxidants have many health benefits if taken before and after cancer treatment, we are cautious about using them during treatment because the potential for diminishing the benefit of the treatment exists. ■

Katrina VB Claghorn, MS, RD

> 66 there is potential that the antioxidant activity of grapeseed may interfere with chemotherapy

Q: *Herbal supplements and chemotherapy.*
Can you take any type of herbal supplements while on
chemotherapy? Is it OK to take Moducare through
chemotherapy?

Because there is so little valid research on the interactions between
herbal supplements and chemotherapy, oncologists and dietitians do not
recommend any herbal-type supplements at all during treatment. Many
herbs can act as blood thinners and antioxidants, for example, which
would be contraindicated during chemotherapy.

Another concern is that since herbal supplements are not regulated
at all in the USA, their purity, quality, and standardization are highly
questionable, not to mention the 'cancer cure' claims they sometimes
make when there is no quality research to substantiate it.

Moducare is one of these supplements. The company that makes it claims
that it has researched its immune-stimulating effects. The company has
done some limited, seemingly valid research (not in the USA however)
on its immune-stimulating effects in AIDS and prostate problems, but no
significant research in cancer. Taking any of these 'immune-enhancing'
supplements is not advised because of the lack of valid research to
support its use, its effectiveness, and its safety.

The most immune-enhancing effects have been seen with a diet, not
supplements, that is high in fruits and vegetables (7–9 servings per day).
The only supplement that is recommended during treatment is a

66 oncologists and dietitians do
not recommend any herbal-type
supplements at all during treatment

standard (Centrum type) multivitamin/mineral. If you have further questions on supplements, including herbals, ask an oncology dietitian, if one is available near you. ■

Ellen Sweeney-Cordes, MS, RD

It is claimed that herbs contain many compounds, which may prevent or treat cancer. These compounds have different properties, some stimulate the immune system, while others may encourage cell breakdown or act as antioxidants. Herbs may be recommended for various conditions, but pain or nausea and vomiting are of greatest interest for cancer patients.

Historically, herbs were used as medicines and it is advised that they be treated with the same caution as you would any drug or medication. When considering herbal therapies you should investigate how they function in your therapy and how they may affect your treatment. It is not recommended that you replace conventional medical treatments with herbs. For example, a herb that has antioxidant properties should be avoided during your chemotherapy or radiation therapy, since there is the possibility that it may reduce the effectiveness of the treatments. There is very little information about safe doses for herbs. It is generally recommended that you follow the dosage information provided on the packaging and avoid excesses.

Always inform your doctor of any herbs you are taking. One major concern with herbal remedies is that you may be self-treating symptoms. This could mask important warning signs from your doctor and cause you to delay alerting your medical team. It is difficult to make broad recommendations on the applicability of herbal remedies due to the lack of clinical trials evaluating them. There are studies in progress that will hopefully shed additional light on the benefits of herbal treatments. ■

Katrina VB Claghorn, MS, RD

66
you should investigate how they
function in your therapy and how
they may affect your treatment

Hydrazine sulfate as a cancer treatment. Can hydrazine sulfate help with cancer pain and does it have any benefit in terms of survival?

For a number of years there has been interest in the use of hydrazine sulfate to combat the cachexia (decreased appetite, wasting) seen in cancer patients. The interest was sparked by a report from the UCLA Medical Center which states that hydrazine sulfate may favorably influence nutritional status and clinical outcome in patients with non-small-cell lung cancer. The initial enthusiasm has been dampened, unfortunately, by three subsequent prospective trials with larger numbers of patients that have shown no benefit from the addition of hydrazine sulfate to standard treatment regimens. In these trials patients received either hydrazine sulfate or placebo (no medication). A study from the Mayo Clinic found no benefit from the use of hydrazine sulfate in 243 patients with non-small-cell lung cancer and 127 patients with advanced colorectal cancer. Similarly, a study from the Scripps Clinic found no benefit of adding hydrazine sulfate to an effective chemotherapy regimen in 291 patients with advanced non-small-cell lung cancer. Thus hydrazine sulfate does not appear to improve survival.

Morphine is used to control symptoms of pain in patients with advanced cancer. Hydrazine sulfate does not control symptoms of pain, and would not be used as a replacement for morphine. ■

James M Metz, MD

66
Hydrazine sulfate does not control symptoms of pain

The macrobiotic diet. My father has metastatic colon cancer. I have been researching different types of therapy, including nutritional therapy. Is the macrobiotic diet safe and has there been a scientific study into it?

The macrobiotic diet is a very restrictive vegetarian diet. As with any diet that limits food choices there is the potential for nutrient deficiencies. Consequently, if you follow the diet you should consult a registered dietitian to make sure you are getting all the nutrients you need (protein, vitamins, and minerals). If deficiencies exist, adjustments can be made to the diet to ensure it is nutritionally complete. Macrobitics is not limited to just foods; it is also a philosophical and lifestyle program that includes exercise and meditation. Thus, going to a macrobiotic school or instructor is generally suggested.

Making dietary and lifestyle changes is difficult enough for a person who is well, but can be a hardship for a sick person such as your father. Also, a plant-based diet may be hard for a person with a gastrointestinal cancer to tolerate. If your father wishes to try the diet you may be able to adjust the regimen to his needs. However, if he is not committed to the diet these issues would only provide more stress and upset.

So far no studies have shown that the macrobiotic diet can cure cancer. However, the National Institutes of Health is studying the diet. Certainly plant-based diets have been shown to have a role in preventing cancer (as well as other chronic diseases) and a person who works at maintaining their nutrition status after a cancer diagnosis may be better able to deal with cancer treatments and generally feel better. ■

Katrina VB Claghorn, MS, RD

66
a plant-based diet may be hard for a person with a gastrointestinal cancer to tolerate

Max Gerson, a German physician, developed the Gerson diet in the 1940s. The diet, which is often referred to as a metabolic diet, was designed to 'stimulate the immune system'. It includes a regimen of cleansing and detoxification combined with a vegetarian diet and supplements. The program has been promoted by Dr Gerson and his followers as a treatment for cancer and other autoimmune diseases.

Dr Gerson believed that autoimmune disorders were the result of chemicals in foods and the environment poisoning the liver. He also proposed that imbalances in dietary sodium and potassium weakened the immune system and deficiencies of oxygen-supplying enzymes contributed to decreased intestinal flora. The diet attempts to correct the problems he perceives to be causes of cancers and other autoimmune disorders.

The diet requires drinking large amounts of fresh, organic fruit and vegetable juices, originally every hour for 13 hours a day. Meals are organic vegetarian and exclude all animal protein as well as oils, salt, nuts, berries, and processed foods. The diet is supplemented with potassium, thyroid, enzymes, B vitamins, vitamin C, and linseed oil. In addition, coffee and castor oil enemas are used to detoxify the liver. Participants in the program are required to discontinue conventional medical therapies. OncoLink strongly opposes this recommendation.

> **"** the regimen's assumptions have not been scientifically validated

To date the regimen's assumptions have not been scientifically validated. However, the Office of Alternative Medicine of the National Institute of Health has been studying the program to determine its effectiveness. While most aspects of the Gerson regimen have no scientific basis, recent research does support the benefits of a low-fat, plant-based diet in preventing cancer.

The most commonly cited problem associated with the program is that it is very restrictive and difficult to follow. It is also expensive, requiring a visit to one of the Gerson centers for initial detoxification and instruction. Preparation of the juices and meals is extremely time consuming, and the organic foods and supplements can be costly. Physical side-effects of the treatment may include severe nausea, vomiting, and abdominal cramps, as well as aches and pains.

OncoLink strongly recommends that you alert your physician if you are considering the Gerson regimen. Again, it is not recommended by our editorial board that you discontinue any conventional medical cancer treatments in favor of this or any other unconventional or alternative treatments. Rather, it is suggested that you speak to your physicians and healthcare team to plan on working complementary treatments into your conventional treatment plan. ■

Katrina VB Claghorn, MS, RD

Vitamin supplements and cancer. *I have been diagnosed with cancer. Should I take vitamin supplements?*

A well-balanced diet should provide all your vitamin and nutrient requirements. However, the side-effects of chemotherapy and radiation therapy can limit your ability to eat well. In addition, the stress of the treatments may increase your nutritional needs. A standard multivitamin will provide the recommended dietary allowances (RDAs) and therefore prevent potential vitamin and mineral deficiencies. However, it is important to note that, while vitamin and mineral deficiencies may have serious health impacts, toxicity from excessive supplementation can also be serious. Consequently, it is recommended that you take no more than five times the RDA of any nutrient. To determine how much you need of any nutrient, refer to the National Research Council's RDA list, or ask your healthcare provider or a registered dietitian. In addition, always tell your doctor about the supplements you are taking, since some are known to adversely impact your treatment. ■

Katrina VB Claghorn, MS, RD

> ❝ it is recommended that you take no more than five times the RDA of any nutrient

Glutamine supplements for rectal cancer. Do you have any information on the use of glutamine powder as a supplement during treatment for rectal cancer?

Glutamine is an amino acid. Generally, the body produces and maintains adequate levels of glutamine, but when the body is under stress deficiencies can occur. Glutamine is the preferred fuel of the fast-growing cells of the gastrointestinal tract and is essential in maintaining the integrity of the mucosal lining.

Many studies have been done on the use of glutamine in cancer treatments, and while these have generally shown a benefit, the results are inconclusive. When used in conjunction with chemotherapy and radiation therapy, glutamine has been found to reduce some side-effects of the treatments, such as mouth sores, diarrhea, and peripheral neuropathy. There are no known drug or nutrient interactions associated with glutamine. However, anybody who restricts their protein intake for medical reasons should avoid glutamine. Glutamine 30 g/day taken in three 10-g doses is the dosage that has been shown to have the most benefit. ■

Katrina VB Claghorn, MS, RD

66 glutamine has been found to reduce some side-effects of the treatments

Blue-green algae. *A friend of mine has recommended I take a supplement called blue-green algae. Will this help my immune system, as it claims?*

Blue-green algae, also called *Spirulina*, is one of many forms of algae used in algae supplement products. Another common form of algae is called *Chlorella*. The blue-green color of *Spirulina* comes from its high chlorophyll and phycocyanin content, which has been studied for potential anti-inflammatory, antioxidant, and antiviral properties. *Spirulina* is a source of protein and some vitamins and minerals, namely iron. However, it is a more expensive protein source than equivalent amounts of dietary sources and it does not take the place of fruits and vegetables in the diet. Although this supplement contains vitamins and minerals, the amounts are unknown. There is not enough scientific research on blue-green algae to recommend it as an immune stimulant. In addition, some *Spirulina* products are not tested for safety, and have been found to be contaminated with microbes and/or heavy metals that can cause liver toxicity. Use of these products is not recommended during any cancer. ■

Ellen Sweeney-Cordes, MS, RD

" Use of these products is not recommended during any cancer

Antioxidant supplements, which would include vitamins A, C, and E, β-carotene, co-enzyme Q10, and minerals such as selenium, may interfere with cancer treatments. The concern is that antioxidants may reduce the oxidizing free radicals created by the treatments and consequently reduce the effectiveness of the therapy. There have been inconclusive studies in this area, but our knowledge about how chemotherapy and radiation therapy work leads us to predict that antioxidants may interfere with therapy.

Food sources of antioxidants are generally safe, since it would be difficult to consume a large enough amount of antioxidants from food sources, such as fruits and vegetables, to negatively impact treatments. A safe supplement to take during therapy is a standard (Centrum-type brand) multivitamin which generally provides a safe amount and balance of nutrients. ■

Katrina VB Claghorn, MS, RD

"
antioxidants may interfere with therapy

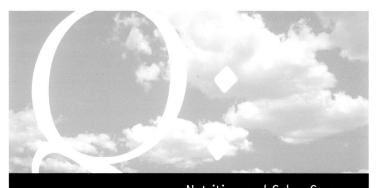

Nutrition and Colon Cancer

Nutrition needs prior to surgery for colon cancer.
My partner is about to undergo surgery for colon cancer.
Are there any recommendations for diet before and after
surgery for colon cancer?

There is no special preoperative diet for colon cancer surgery. The most
important thing is to consume adequate calories and protein to maintain
one's weight so that the patient is not nutritionally depleted going into
surgery. It is even beneficial to gain some weight prior to surgery if there
has been unintentional weight loss leading up to it. There should not be
any limits placed on the patient's diet at this time unless the doctor has
indicated otherwise. ■

Ellen Sweeney-Cordes, MS, RD

66
There should not be any limits placed
on the patient's diet at this time

Q: *Diabetes management with chemotherapy and radiation. My 87-year-old Dad has just been diagnosed with colon cancer. He has indigestion every day now, even though he is on a low-fat diet. He is also a recovering stroke patient, with hypertension and insulin diabetes. He starts chemotherapy and radiation soon. How will the side-effects of chemotherapy and radiation therapy affect his diabetes problems, and how do I manage his food intake and blood sugar levels?*

Depending on the type of chemotherapy drugs and the radiation he receives, your father could experience several side-effects. These side-effects may include nausea, loss of appetite, change in the taste of foods, constipation, and/or diarrhea. Any side-effects that end up affecting the amount he eats can obviously affect his blood sugar levels. If he does not have a loss of appetite and is able to eat normally, then he would continue to treat his diabetes with his current insulin regimen. If his appetite is poor through treatment, it becomes more important for him to get his calorie and protein needs met for weight and protein store maintenance than to follow a diabetic diet. Diabetic patients' diets are liberalized during cancer treatment and these patients are allowed to eat differently during treatment, especially if their appetite is poor. It becomes more important to maintain weight in order to prevent nutritional compromise during treatment. Typically, physicians will adjust oral blood sugar medication or insulin regimens to compensate for the diet changes through treatment. It will be important to track his blood sugars daily to

> 66 Diabetic patients' diets are liberalized during cancer treatment

watch for possible treatment- or eating-related effects. If his sugar levels drop or increase during treatment it is recommended that you contact his primary care physician for insulin adjustments and instruction.

With indigestion, foods containing caffeine, alcohol, and peppermint, in addition to acidic foods (citrus juices and tomato products) and fried foods should be avoided. The diet should not be overly restricted, however, because of indigestion. You may want to consider consulting your father's primary care or oncology physician for medication to help control indigestion.

During cancer treatment dietitians will encourage patients to avoid low-fat products. For example, using whole milk rather than skim milk, regular ice cream, margarine, or butter is recommended to get extra calories when appetite and intake are low. Basically, whatever works food wise is appropriate until the treatment is over and the patient's appetite returns.

Other good high-calorie and protein sources to include in your father's diet (if solid food intake decreases) are liquid supplements such as Ensure Plus® or Boost Plus®. There are also liquid supplements that are specially formulated for diabetics, such as Glucerna® and Choice®. These are readily available in supermarkets and drugstores. In addition, these are good liquid sources of nutrients after a stroke if his swallowing or eating of solid foods has been affected. Considering your father's age and medical history, I would recommend that you ask for a consultation with an oncology dietitian where he is being treated (if available) to assess his calorie and protein needs and provide individual nutrition counseling. ◼

Ellen Sweeney-Cordes, MS, RD

Q: *Nutritional supplements for low blood counts.*
Are there any supplements or foods that can help raise a
white blood cell count that is too low in order to allow the
next round of chemotherapy? Is there any nutrition advice
for a patient on Neupogen?

There are no supplements or specific foods known to increase white blood cell counts. People often confuse iron supplementation with low white blood cell count. Iron supplementation is only appropriate with low red blood cells. The Neupogen medication helps increase white blood cell production. There are no nutrition recommendations with Neupogen, since it does not affect digestion or interact with any food.

However, when white blood cells are low, a patient is at higher risk for infection, so avoidance of uncooked raw fruits and vegetables is important during this time. Raw, uncooked fruits and vegetables may potentially harbor bacteria. Well-cooked vegetables or canned fruits are fine to have. All in all, the best way to insure good immune function and white blood cell production is to eat a well-balanced diet with adequate calories to maintain weight and adequate protein through treatment. A person usually needs 1.2–1.5 g of protein for each kilogram of body weight and 13–15 calories for each pound of body weight. If appetite is poor, then supplement with Boost® or Ensure® liquid supplements for additional calories and protein to maintain weight and protein stores. For further concerns, ask to speak with a registered dietitian at your cancer center. ∎

Ellen Sweeney-Cordes, MS, RD

> " avoidance of uncooked raw fruits and vegetables is important

Maintaining your nutrition status during the course of cancer treatment is a goal shared by the medical team. However, the side-effects of the therapies as well as the disease itself can make it difficult to take in enough nutrients. Some of the symptoms that can cause decreased nutrient intake include a loss of appetite, difficulty swallowing, or inflammation of mucous membranes in your mouth. Furthermore, because the cancer or the cancer therapies can increase your metabolic rate, your body may need more nutrients. While the best way to insure adequate nutrition is through a diet that includes a variety of foods, there may be times when you are unable to meet your nutrition needs from food alone and nutrition supplements can help fill the gap.

Most of the traditional nutritional supplements resemble a milk shake, and come in a wide variety of flavors. Newer more popular products are also available in a high calorie or Aplus® version. If these high-calorie products are too sweet they can be thinned with milk to decrease the thickness and the sweetness. Some products resemble a fruit drink supplement (mix this drink with ginger ale to make a punch) for those who do not like the milk shake version. This fruit-based supplement, as well as the low-lactose drinks, are indicated for patients experiencing diarrhea. Instant Breakfast® mixes can be purchased in the grocery store and can be used as a supplement. These supplements are added to milk products to provide extra protein and calories. While they may not be as nutritionally complete as the commercial supplements, these Instant Breakfast® mixes are much less expensive.

> " there may be times when you are unable to meet your nutrition needs from food alone and nutrition supplements can help fill the gap

Nutrition supplements can play an important role in minimizing the wasting cachexia so often seen during cancer therapy. Aggressive use of supplements along with education on symptom management can help prevent malnutrition and may improve tolerance to treatment. With supplements now available in bars and puddings as well as beverages, you should be able to find a supplement that you like and can include in your meal plan. The following is a recipe for a supplemental shake:

- mix one packet of Carnation Instant Breakfast® into one 8-oz (0.25-liter) can of a nutritional supplement

- blend in one to two scoops of ice cream.

This drink provides about 500 calories and 20 g of protein, depending on the supplement used. ■

Katrina VB Claghorn, MS, RD

Patients with radiation enteritis are generally recommended to follow a low-fiber, low-lactose, and low-fat diet. Sometimes a gluten restriction may be needed. Because the diet can be so restrictive it is best to meet with a registered dietitian who can instruct you on foods that can be tolerated and develop a meal plan that will provide all your nutrition needs.

However, most patients tolerate a regular diet of six small frequent meals better than three large meals. The small meals need to be nutritionally complete, containing adequate protein and calories. A general goal is that each small meal should contain no less than 300 calories and at least 10 g of protein. If weight loss continues, add nutrition supplements (e.g. Carnation Instant Breakfast® (made with Lactaid milk), Boost®, or Ensure®). There is a wonderful product called Scandishake® that provides 600 calories per 8-oz (0.25-liter) serving, but it has to be ordered from your pharmacist.

The main problem during periods of enteritis is significant diarrhea. Rice, apple sauce, and bananas are the foods that may help with diarrhea. Adding pectin powder to your food (but start with small amounts) may also decrease diarrhea.

Some helpful resources are:

" recommended to follow a low-fiber, low-lactose, and low-fat diet

■ The National Cancer Institute's booklet *Eating Hints* (US Department of Health and Human Services, Public Health Service, National Institutes of Health, Bethesda, MD, 1997) is a good source of information on symptom management, diet, and nutrition for people undergoing cancer treatments. It also contains recipes that are high in nutritional value and are delicious.

■ Daniel W Nixon, *The Cancer Recovery Eating Plan* (Three Rivers Press, New York, 1996). ■

Katrina VB Claghorn, MS, RD

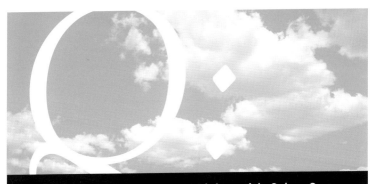

Living with Colon Cancer

Q: *Nutritional changes following substantial colon resection. I am looking for information about changes in bowel habits, changes in diet, other practical hints, tips, etc., after substantial colon resection following surgery involving two synchronous cancers with many polyps. The rectum will remain intact and colostomy is not anticipated.*

Following a colon resection I would recommend a low-fiber, low-lactose, and low-fat diet. However, as the bowel recovers, fiber should be gradually reintroduced and regular dairy foods should be tolerated. In addition, make sure you are including high-protein foods to help your body rebuild.

As for changes in bowel habits, both diarrhea and constipation may be experienced. If diarrhea is a problem, avoid high-lactose foods and include rice, bananas and apple sauce, as well as making sure you drink plenty of fluids. For constipation, increase your intake of fiber (fruits, vegetables, and whole grains) and drink plenty of fluids.

Following surgery you may need supplements of vitamin B_{12}, but discuss this with your doctor. ▪

Katrina VB Claghorn, MS, RD

“ make sure you are including high-protein foods to help your body rebuild

Q: *Increase in carcinoembryonic antigen (CEA) after colon surgery. My husband had a colostomy almost 3 years ago. Right after surgery his CEA level was 0.8 or 0.9. His most recent CEA is 11. He has been on Lipitor and Moducare and radiologic tests have been scheduled. Could either of these drugs or other factors cause a high CEA level, and does an elevated reading necessarily indicate cancer growth?*

The value of determining CEA levels for follow-up after resection of a colon cancer has been controversial. Many have advocated it, while others have felt that it adds little to patient care. The idea is that an elevation would detect an earlier cancer recurrence, allowing therapy to be initiated and thus resulting in a better outcome. Data are available to support both positions.

A CEA of 11, while elevated, falls into that intermediate range that is difficult to interpret. It has risen since the last one, and evaluating the situation with radiologic tests to look for recurrent cancer is wise. If these do not indicate any tumor, you may be able to follow the CEA level closely to see if it continues to rise. I am unaware if either of the medications you mentioned can cause an elevation in CEA levels. The companies that make those drugs may be able to answer this question better than I. As you may know, certain behaviors, such as smoking, can raise CEA levels unrelated to any cancer. ■

Timothy C Hoops, MD

> " certain behaviors, such as smoking, can raise CEA levels unrelated to any cancer

Q: *Rising carcinoembryonic antigen(CEA) level after surgery. I am a 45-year-old, non-smoking male who at 41 was diagnosed with colorectal cancer. My CEA at diagnosis was 57. I had chemotherapy and radiation therapy followed by surgery. Postoperatively I was treated with 5-fluorouracil (5-FU) for 3 months. Ten months after surgery a tumor was detected in my liver and was removed. My CEA level at the time of liver tumor detection was 8.2. Over the last year my CEA level has slowly risen, the most recent value being 21, which jumped from 13. I have had repeated computed tomography (CT) scans and nuclear studies which have shown nothing. The last colonoscopy was 10 months ago. I find it hard to believe nothing can be found. Any suggestions?*

This is a difficult clinical scenario. As you know, we use CEA levels to point out that there could be recurrence of the cancer. It is certainly reassuring that your recent CT scans and nuclear studies have not identified a recurrence of your tumor. It would be important to ensure that there is no spread to your lungs, as isolated pulmonary metastases can be resected for cure. This is similar to your liver operation. I would encourage you to go ahead and seek a second opinion with an oncologist who specializes in this area. ■

James D Lewis, MD, MSCE

66 seek a second opinion with an oncologist who specializes in this area

Exercises for pelvic radiation fibrosis. One of the
physiotherapists in our agency has been asked to develop
an exercise program for a lady who has radiation fibrosis in
her abdomen and pelvis. She had her radiation treatments
about 4–5 months ago. What factors should the
physiotherapist consider?

Radiation changes the pliability of muscles, fascia, and skin. These
changes often occur weeks to months after radiation has ended. It is
beneficial to provide patients with a prophylactic stretching program while
undergoing radiation therapy and after it has ended to help avoid fibrosis.

Once fibrosis occurs, you can use many of the deep techniques used in
the general population. Ideas include massage, stretching, and joint
mobilization. In addition, many therapists have found myofascial release
techniques to be quite effective. It is also important to address any issues
of pelvic pain, lymphedema, incontinence, and pain with intercourse, as
these may also be side-effects of radiation to the pelvic region.

There are some relative contraindications to deep techniques after radiation:

■ do not use deep techniques over acutely irradiated skin

■ do not use deep techniques over any open wounds or fragile skin

■ do not use electrotherapies without discussion with the physician. ■

Lora Packel, MS, PT

66 you can use many of the deep
techniques used in the general
population

In the early 1990s a study was done in which about 1500 patients who had undergone polypectomy were divided randomly into two groups. One group had follow-up colonoscopies at 1 and 3 years, while the other group had a repeat colonoscopy at 3 years only. The study demonstrated that there was no difference between the two groups in the number of recurrent polyps or cancers found. This changed the practice of gastroenterology from yearly follow-up colonoscopy, which had been the standard, to colonoscopy every 3 years.

The same researchers have shown that if there were fewer than three polyps and they were very small, it was probably safe to wait even 5 years for the next procedure. These data support what is known about the biology of the development of cancer. In most, if not all, cases cancers develop from adenomatous polyps. The process of going from normal tissue to polyp to cancer is quite long, extending from 10 to 15 years, and possibly even longer. Thus, the longer interval between colonoscopies after removal of a polyp is safe and reduces the discomfort and small risk associated with these procedures.

It may benefit your father to have a colonoscopy no earlier than 3 years after the last, unless there was some specific finding that warranted an earlier procedure. ■

Timothy C Hoops, MD

> **"** The process of going from normal tissue to polyp to cancer is quite long, extending from 10 to 15 years, and possibly even longer

This is a very important question that has not been well answered. Keep your eyes open and you may see information in the news. At a minimum, all patients with colon cancer should speak with their physician to determine whether or not they may have a familial cancer syndrome. Patients with a familial cancer syndrome are clearly at increased risk for many other types of cancers, as may be some of their relatives. Lastly, persons who have had one colon cancer are at increased risk for another colon cancer, and should be closely monitored in a cancer surveillance program. Consider enrolling in the OncoLink/National Colorectal Cancer Research Alliance colorectal cancer prevention database (see the end of this book). ■

James D Lewis, MD, MSCE

> **"** persons who have had one colon cancer are at increased risk for another colon cancer

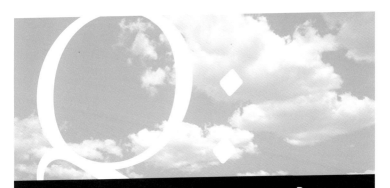

Resources

FAMILIAL ADENOMATOUS POLYPOSIS

To learn more about surgical options for familial adenomatous polyposis (FAP), visit the Mt. Sinai Hospital website from Toronto, Canada:

http://www.mtsinai.on.ca/familialgican/FAPEnglish/fap7.html

To learn more about the ileoanal anastomosis procedure and support see:

http://www.jpouch.org

To find a genetic counselor in your area see:

http://www.cancer.gov/search/genetics_services

To learn more about cancer family registries see:

http://epi.grants.cancer.gov/CFR

To calculate your cancer risk see:

http://www.yourcancerrisk.harvard.edu/index.htm

To learn more about cancer family research supported by the NCCRA see:

http://www.nccra.com/clinical_research/index.htm

BOOKS AND VIDEO REVIEWS ON COLORECTAL CANCER

Lorraine Johnson 1999 Colon & rectal cancer: a comprehensive guide for patients and families. Patient-Centered Guides, O'Reilly, Sebastopol, CA. ISBN 1565926331   This book conveys accurate and reliable information in an easily readable format. The book is well planned and organized to follow the path and experiences of colorectal cancer patients. Survivor stories are tactfully incorporated throughout the book, and these both emphasize important points and bring a personal flavor to the book. The reader will gain a strong knowledge base on colorectal cancer that will help them interact with their healthcare provider.

A. Richard Adrouny 2002 Understanding colon cancer. University Press of Mississippi, Jackson, MS. ISBN 1578064732.   Dr Richard Adrouny is the director of medical oncology at the community hospital of Los Gatos-Saratoga and a clinical assistant professor of medicine at Stanford University School of Medicine. This book provides the reader with patient-friendly information, covering topics such as genetics, diagnosis, staging, prognosis, and treatment. The book also includes a chapter on the future of colon cancer screening and treatment.

Bernard Levin 1999 The American Cancer Society: colorectal cancer. Villard Books, New York. ISBN 0679778136. This is an important reference for anyone interested in the prevention and treatment of these cancers. The author is the Chair of the American Cancer Society's National Advisory Task Force on Colorectal Cancer and Vice President for Cancer Prevention at the University of Texas MD Anderson Cancer Center. The book is an excellent resource for anyone interested in the prevention, screening, and treatment of colorectal cancer. The book emphasizes prevention and early detection, and therefore provides important information for everyone, not just the cancer patient.

Paul Miskovitz and Marian Betancourt 1997 What to do if you get colon cancer: a specialist helps you take charge and make informed choices. Wiley, New York. ISBN 0471159840. Dr Miskovitz is a Clinical Associate Professor of Medicine at Cornell University Medical College, and an Associate Attending Physician at the New York Hospital, and Ms Betancourt is a writer. For people with colon cancer, this guide can answer questions about treatment options, as well as provide practical advice on every aspect of recovery and how to get back to life. The book is written in a caring, patient-friendly style, and will help the reader gain a basic knowledge in order to make treatment decisions and better communicate with their physician.

Judith McKay and Nancee Hirano 1998 The chemotherapy & radiation therapy survival guide. New Harbinger, Oakland, CA. ISBN 1572240709. Both authors are seasoned oncology nurses at the Alta Bates Comprehensive Cancer Center in Berkeley, California. The nurses draw from their first-hand experiences with patients to explain chemotherapy, radiation therapy, intravenous therapy, and the side-effects associated with them. The book offers chapters on relaxation, stress reduction, and the mind–body connection.

Elaine Magee 2001 Tell me what to eat to help prevent colon cancer. New Page Books, Franklin Lakes, NJ. ISBN 156414514X. This book begins with an overview of colon cancer in patient-friendly terminology. Readers gain a better understanding of what colon cancer is and what actions they can take to help prevent it. The author is a dietician, and answers questions about colon cancer prevention through dietary changes. You will find a host of specific recommendations about what to eat, what to avoid, and how to incorporate these changes in your lifestyle. The book also includes dozens of healthful, practical, and tasty recipes, focusing on fiber and power produce items.

Barbara Barrie and Otis W Brawley 1999 Don't die of embarrassment: life after colostomy and other adventures. Fireside Books, Forest City, NJ. ISBN 0684846241.   Academy Award nominated actress Barbara Barrie began writing this book after she was diagnosed with rectal cancer in 1994 while acting in the television mini-series *Scarlett*. The book takes the reader through Barbara's journey of symptoms, diagnosis, surgery, radiation therapy, chemotherapy, and life with a colostomy. It is a candid view of her experiences with her family, friends, and the medical profession. The ups and downs of living with a colostomy are discussed from a very personal viewpoint.

Barbara Dorr Mullen and Kerry Anne McGinn 1992 The ostomy book: living comfortably with colostomies, ileostomies, and urostomies. Bull Publishing, Boulder, CO. ISBN 0923521127.   This book is written with the first-hand experience of a 'colostomate' and an endostomal therapist. Half of the royalties generated from book sales are donated to the United Ostomy Association. The book covers topics such as descriptions of different types of ostomies and surgeries, traveling with an ostomy, considering work situations, remaining active with exercise, children with ostomies, sex, and emotional adjustments.

Kathy Foley-Bolch, Michelle Fallon Kasouf, Barbara Kupfer, and W. Brian Sweeney 2000 Yes we can! Advice on traveling yes with an ostomy and tips for everyday living. Chandler House Press, Worcester, MA. ISBN 1886284598.   Barbara Kupfer, Kathy Foley-Bolch, and Michelle Fallon Kasouf have all had ostomy surgery. Dr W Brain Sweeney was formerly Chief of Colorectal Surgery at the University of Massachusetts Hospital in Worcester, Massachusetts. This pocket-sized guide covers an enormous range of useful information and details every issue that may arise when traveling with an ostomy, such as what to bring, dietary considerations, ways of travel, toileting, emergency situations, and tips for physically challenged people. At the end of the book, six comprehensive appendices list worldwide resources, international organizations, suppliers, and even key words and phases translated into 11 languages.

Paul Ruggieri 2001 Colon and rectal cancer: a patient's guide to treatment. Addicus Books, Omaha, NE. ISBN 1886039518.   The author is Chief of the Department of Surgery at St. Anne's Hospital in Fall River,

Massachusetts. He specializes in thyroid and minimally invasive surgery. He is the author of *The Surgery Handbook – A Guide to Understanding your Operation*. This book about colon and rectal cancer covers topics such as symptoms and risk factors, prevention, diagnostic testing, staging, and various treatments and how they work.

GENERAL RESOURCES: INTERNET SITES

American Cancer Society: Colon and Rectum Cancer   The ACS website provides information for patients and health professionals on all types of cancer. Information is available on ACS programs throughout the country. Information is also available in Spanish.

URL: http://www.cancer.org

American Society of Colon and Rectal Surgeons   This site has a section of 'patient brochures' that addresses some issues related to colon cancer. The site also allows you to search for a colon and rectal surgeon in your area.

URL: http://www.fascrs.org

American Society for Gastrointestinal Endoscopy   This is the website of the professional society for gastroenterologists. There is information on colonoscopy and other gastrointestinal procedures, in both English and Spanish, as well as general information on colon cancer.

URL: http://www.asge.org

Cancer Backup   A web-based resource from the UK with a mission to give cancer patients and their families the up-to-date information, practical advice, and support they need to reduce the fear and uncertainty of cancer.

URL: http://www.cancerbaccup.org

CANCERLIT: Gastrointestinal Cancers   The National Cancer Institute's CANCERLIT database includes citations and abstracts on such topics as screening and prevention of digestive cancers, therapy of colorectal cancer and diagnosis and pathogenesis of gastric cancer.

URL: http://www.cancer.gov/search/cancer_literature/
search_cancerlittopic.aspx?key=19&topic=Gastrointestinal+Cancers

Cancer Research Foundation of America   This organization promotes prevention and early detection of certain cancers through scientific research and education. The site provides information on the programs they support and recent news.

URL: http://www.preventcancer.org/index.cfm

Colon Cancer Alliance This is a support, education, and advocacy organization for patients. It provides survivor stories, information on clinical trials, and an online chat service. Resources available include disease information, a question and answer forum, news, current activities, and screening facts.

URL: http://www.ccalliance.org

Colorectal Cancer Association of Canada This site provides information on the educational and support activities for patients organized by the association. The site provides news, resources, and clinical trial information. The information is also available in French.

URL: http://www.ccac-accc.ca

Dad's Colon Cancer Pages This site provides a thorough collection of links to other sites, which has been developed and maintained by the son of a colon cancer patient. Information ranges from the very basic to detailed in the areas of research, nutrition, gene therapy, surgery, and diagnosis. The site is updated frequently.

URL: http://members.tripod.com/~cancer49

Harvard Center for Cancer Prevention: Your Cancer Risk This interactive website offers questionnaires about various types of cancer, calculates an estimated cancer risk, and gives personalized tips for prevention. The site also offers information on types of cancer, discussions of risk factors, and screening tests.

URL: http://www.yourcancerrisk.harvard.edu

InTouchLive.com: Colorectal Cancer This is an online version of the magazine *Colorectal Cancer*. It provides extensive information about cancer. Information specific to colon cancer can be found under the CANCERS menu, and then GASTROINTESTINAL CANCERS. Topics include news, diagnosis, staging, treatment, and prevention.

URL: http://intouchlive.com

Johns Hopkins GI – Colon Cancer Resources This site is produced by

Johns Hopkins Department of Gastroenterology. It has information on diagnosis, staging, treatment, hereditary syndromes, and more. The information can also be translated into Spanish and Chinese.

URL: http://hopkins-gi.org/pages/latin/templates/index.cfm

MD Anderson Cancer Center   This site provides information on colon cancer, patient support, news, clinical trials and other resources. Also included is a section on hereditary colon cancers.

URL: http://www.mdanderson.org/Diseases/Colorectal

MEDLINEplus Health Information: Colorectal Cancer   The National Library of Medicine offers links to other websites for news stories, clinical trials, diagnosis, screening, treatment and research findings. The site also offers glossaries, statistics, and information specific to seniors and women. Some information is also available in Spanish.

URL: http://www.nlm.nih.gov/medlineplus/colorectalcancer.html

National Cancer Institute (NCI) PDQ: Colon Cancer   The purpose of this site is to provide physicians with guidelines for the treatment of colon cancer. The PDQ offers a general overview of the disease, including staging and treatment options.

NCI/PDQ® Patient Statement: Colon Cancer

NCI/PDQ® Physician Statement: Colon Cancer

NCI/PDQ® Physician Statement: Prevention of Colorectal Cancer

URL: http://www.cancer.gov/cancer_information/doc_pdq.aspx?version= provider&viewid=2cfe2c5f-9e61–4026-a62e-939e818fd165

National Colorectal Cancer Action Campaign   The Centers for Disease Control and Prevention (CDC) details its action campaign at this site. Information is provided on the 'Screen for Life' program, which is dedicated to educating the public on the importance of having regular colorectal screening tests. Links to related resources are included.

URL: http://www.cdc.gov/cancer/screenforlife

National Colorectal Cancer Research Alliance   The NCCRA is dedicated to the eradication of colon cancer by harnessing the power of celebrity to promote education, fundraising, research, and early medical screening. Founded by Katie Couric, Lily Tartikoff, and the

Entertainment Industry Foundation, their website offers facts on colorectal cancer, screening information, a clinical trials resource center, and related links.

URL: http://www.nccra.org

National Surgical Adjuvant Breast and Bowel Project   The NSABP is a group that performs clinical trials in the areas of breast and colon cancer. The site provides a description of their trials, news and updates of ongoing trials, contact information, a list of references, and details of future meetings.

URL: http://www.nsabp.pitt.edu

New York Online Access to Health (NOAH): Colon, Rectal, and Anal Cancer   This website, maintained by four New York Library Associations, includes information on colon cancer screening, diagnosis, treatment, clinical trials and side-effect management. The site also offers information in Spanish.

URL: http://www.noah-health.org/english/illness/cancer/cancer.html

OncoLink   OncoLink was founded in 1994 by University of Pennsylvania cancer specialists with a mission to help cancer patients, families, healthcare professionals and the general public get accurate cancer-related information at no charge. Through OncoLink you can get comprehensive information about specific types of cancer, updates on cancer treatments, and news about research advances. We update the information every day and provide information at various levels, from introductory to in depth. If you are interested in learning about cancer, you will benefit from visiting OncoLink.

OncoLink Editorial Board, Abramson Cancer Center of the University of Pennsylvania, 3400 Spruce Street – 2 Donner, Philadelphia, PA 19104, USA

E-mail: editors@oncolink.com

URL: http://www.oncolink.upenn.edu

United Ostomy Association   The UOA is a non-profit organization providing information and support for patients. The website offers information about ostomies, local chapters, conferences, insurance issues, and discussion boards. The UOA local chapters provide a service through which certified visitors are made available to patients in need.

URL: http://www.uoa.org

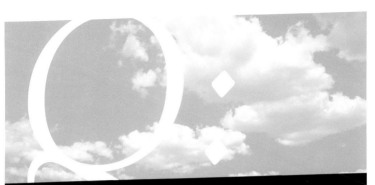

References

A guide for families: familial adenomatous polyposis. Familial Gastrointestinal Registry, Mount Sinai Hospital, Toronto Canada. URL: http://www.mtsinai.on.ca/familialgican/default.htm

American Cancer Society 2001 Statistics. URL: http://www.cancer.org

Hampel H, Peltomaki P 2000 Hereditary colorectal cancer: risk assessment and management. Clinical Genetics 58:89–97

Lal G, Gallinger S 2000 Familial adenomatous polyposis. Seminars in Surgical Oncology 18:314–323

Lenhard RE, Osteen RT, Gansler T (eds) 2001 The American Cancer Society's clinical oncology. The American Cancer Society, Atlanta, GA

CancerNet, a service of the National Cancer Institute. Genetics, causes, risk factors, prevention of colon and rectal cancer. URL: http://www.cancer.gov/cancerinfo

Vasen HF, Watson P, Mecklin JP, et al 1999 New clinical criteria for hereditary nonpolyposis colorectal cancer (HNPCC, Lynch syndrome) proposed by the International Collaborative Group on HNPCC. Gastroenterology 116:1453–1456

Yarbro CH, Frogge MH, Goodman M, et al (eds) 2001 Cancer nursing: principles and practice. Jones and Bartlett, Boston, MA

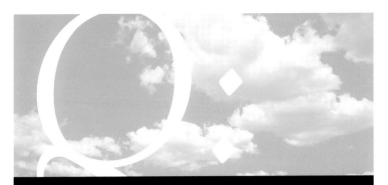

It is key for cancer patients to keep a record of all the physicians involved in their care. Since most patients are treated with more than one therapy for cancer, there may be many physicians involved. Keeping an up-to-date list allows the patient to reference their physicians quickly. It is also important that all your physicians know who else is involved in your care. Notes about your condition can be sent to other physicians if you provide the names and addresses. This allows for care to flow smoothly, since all your physicians are informed regularly on your progress. The following chart can serve as an important guide. This list can be copied and handed to each of your physicians to place with your records. Most patients are overwhelmed by the number of appointments that are scheduled for their cancer care. Keeping an appointment note is an easy way to make sure that you do not miss any of your scheduled visits. Make sure to add your next visit to the appointment book before leaving your physician's office and use the notes section to write down any important information discussed at the appointment or questions for your next visit.

Physician name	Address	Phone/fax numbers	Specialty	Next appointment Date/time	Notes

It is very important for cancer patients to keep a list of all the medications they are currently taking. This includes herbs, vitamins, over-the-counter remedies, and unconventional medical treatments.

An important note. Sometimes patients feel uncomfortable discussing these treatments with their doctor. It is important to have an open dialogue with the physicians responsible for your care. Many of these therapies can have interactions with conventional medications. They may also cause side-effects that could wrongly be attributed to either the disease process or conventional treatments. For these reasons, your healthcare provider should be notified about these treatments.

It is important to carry the list at all times. Cancer patients may be under the care of a number of different physicians and not all the doctors may know what others have prescribed. Significant interactions can occur with some medicines and supplements, and your doctor needs to consider these before prescribing any new medication.

It is important to list the name of each medication or supplement, the dose in milligrams, and the frequency with which it is taken. The doctor who prescribed the medication and the date medication started should also be listed. Use the following chart to document any medications, over-the-counter remedies, vitamins, herbs, or other non-conventional treatments that are being utilized.

Name of medicine	Dose (mg)	Frequency of taking	Physician who prescribed	Date started	Reason for medicine

CHEMOTHERAPY HISTORY

During some part of their treatment course, many cancer patients receive chemotherapy. Chemotherapy is normally given in 'cycles'. Each cycle lasts, on average, 3–4 weeks. Patients may receive a number of different chemotherapy agents in combination or at different times during their treatment. It is important that all physicians involved in the patient's care are aware of the various drugs being used. There can be important side-effects, interactions with medications, and interactions with other therapies. The following chart will help sort out this important information:

Name of chemotherapy	Date cycle started	Cycle number	Medical oncologist	Notes Side-effects

RADIATION THERAPY HISTORY

A considerable number of cancer patients will receive radiation therapy. The amount of radiation therapy given is restricted over a person's lifetime. It is important that your radiation oncologist is aware of *any* radiation that may have been delivered in the past. Patients should keep a record of when they are treated, the location on the body treated, the total dose delivered, and the name of the radiation oncologist responsible for delivering the treatments. Utilize the following chart to register any treatments with radiation therapy:

Date of radiation	Body part treated	Total dose	Radiation oncologist	Notes Side-effects

PAST HOSPITALIZATIONS/SURGERIES

Make a list of any hospital admissions and/or surgeries. Make sure the date, the reason for hospitalization or the type of surgery, the name of hospital, the physician, and any complications are included. Thinking about any hospitalizations or surgeries will help you and your physician identify past medical issues. Use the following chart to help sort out this important information. Do not forget to list the following procedures if they have been performed: tonsillectomy, gall bladder removal, appendectomy, and removal of skin cancers. These all count as surgery. Note any complications that you have experienced from the surgery.

Date	Reason for hospitalization/ type of surgery	Name of hospital	Physician	Complications

Many cancer patients will have many radiologic studies done during the work-up and follow-up of a specific cancer. These studies may include x-rays, computed tomography (CT) scans, magnetic resonance imaging (MRI) scans, ultrasound studies, and bone scans, to name just a few. It is important to keep a list of all studies that have been performed. These studies may be done at different facilities. It is important for the patient to provide a list of the tests completed and the locations at which the studies were done. This helps each of your physicians to obtain the results of these procedures. Always follow-up on the results of each of your tests with the physician who ordered it. Do not just assume the results are OK if you do not hear anything. Utilize the following chart to help keep track of each study that has been performed:

Name of procedure	Date completed	Location of study	Phone number	Physician ordering study	Discussed results (Yes/No)

FAMILY HISTORY OF CANCER

Your physician will ask you about any other family members who have developed cancer. There are many cancers that have genetic links. Take time to think about parents, grandparents, and siblings who may have had a diagnosis of cancer. Also note the approximate age at which these family members were diagnosed with cancer. This information may help your physician decide if genetic testing or counseling should be performed.

Name of family member	Relationship	Type of cancer	Age of diagnosis

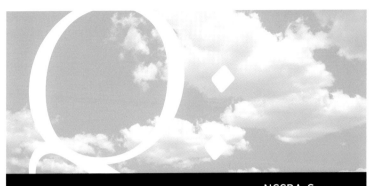

The following introduction, database consent form, and survey form can be found at the following web addresses:

- Introduction: http://www.oncolink.com/nccra/survey_intro.cfm
- Database consent form: http://www.oncolink.com/nccra/consent.cfm
- OncoLink/NCCRA Survey: https://webserv1.iaccelerate.com/oncolink/survey.html

For contact details see p. 177.

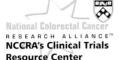

National Colorectal Cancer
R E S E A R C H   A L L I A N C E™
**NCCRA's Clinical Trials
Resource Center**

OncoLink/NCCRA Colorectal Cancer Survey Introduction

This confidential survey was developed by cancer experts as an interactive way to help our leading scientists study families with a history of colorectal cancer. Although the survey contains several questions about you and your family, it should only take about 10 minutes of your time. Your answers may help the NCCRA study the risk factors associated with colorectal cancer and identify potential preventive and treatment therapies. We assure you that your answers will remain on a secure server. Only the principal investigators and participating researchers in the clinical trials approved by the NCCRA scientific advisory board will have access to your information in order to determine your initial eligibility for their particular trial.

After you complete the survey, your name will be entered into a national registry. NCCRA scientists will use the information you volunteer to determine your eligibility for research studies called clinical trials that will help us find ways to prevent and treat this potentially devastating disease. If you are eligible for a trial you will be contacted by one of the NCCRA research scientists.

Remember that your eligibility for these trials is based upon the answers you provide today. If your health history changes, please visit again and repeat the survey to update our registry.

So, let's get started! In less than 10 minutes you can help us make progress toward conquering colorectal cancer.

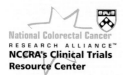

National Colorectal Cancer
R E S E A R C H   A L L I A N C E™
**NCCRA's Clinical Trials
Resource Center**

OncoLink/NCCRA Database Consent

I understand:

- That I am registering into a database for consideration of involvement in future clinical trials.

- That these trials will be used for the possible prevention and treatment of colorectal cancer or study of familial risk factors.

- They are endorsed by the NCCRA.

- That any information I submit will be secure.

- That this secure information will be used to determine my eligibility to participate in clinical trials for colorectal cancer prevention and treatment.

- That submission of information to this database in no way obligates me to participate in any clinical trials.

- That I may withdraw from participation in this database at any time for any reason.

I will allow:

- Representatives of the NCCRA to contact me regarding my eligibility to participate in future clinical trials.

- Representatives of the NCCRA to use the information I provide for an unlimited period of time.

If you have any questions about this study, consent form, or survey please feel free to contact us at editors@oncolink.com.

Signed   *Date*

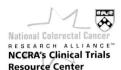

National Colorectal Cancer
RESEARCH ALLIANCE™
**NCCRA's Clinical Trials
Resource Center**

OncoLink/NCCRA Colorectal Cancer Survey

Questions marked with an asterisk are required.

* First Name: [   ]

* Last Name: [   ]

* Date of Birth: [   ] / [   ] / [   ] (mm/dd/yy, ex. 03/08/63)

* Gender: [-   ]

* Address: [   ]

[   ]

* City: [   ]

* State: [   ]   * Zip code: [   ]

* Home Phone: [   ]

Work Phone: [   ]

Can we call you at work? ○ Yes ○ No

Fax: [   ]

Email: [   ]

How did you find out about the OncoLink/NCCRA colorectal
cancer research database?

[   ]

Ethnic/racial background: Self

[   ]

Biological mother:

[   ]

Biological father:

[   ]

What best describes your religious affiliation? (Please give only one response)

[   ]

What is your current marital status?

[   ]

Have you ever been screened for colon cancer? O Yes O No

Has a doctor ever told you that you had any of the following conditions?

Condition	Age at diagnosis
☐ Colon polyps	[ ]
☐ Inflammatory bowel disease	[ ]
☐ Ulcerative colitis	[ ]
☐ Crohn's disease	[ ]
☐ Familial Adenomatous Polyposis (FAP)	[ ]
☐ Hereditary Non-Polyposis Colon Cancer (HPNCC)	[ ]

Is your mother living? O Yes O No

Is your father living? O Yes O No

Number of living brothers: [ ]

Number of living sisters: [ ]

* Have you ever been diagnosed with colorectal cancer or cancer of any kind?

O Yes O No

If yes, has the colorectal cancer spread to other organs (eg, liver or lung)?

O Yes O No Organs: [   ]

If you have colorectal cancer that has spread, how are you doing in terms of your ability to function:

O Fully active, able to carry on all usual activities without restriction

O Restricted in physically strenuous activity but able to walk and able to carry out light housework or office work

O Confined to bed or chair for 50% or more of waking hours

O Totally confined to bed or chair

Have you had chemotherapy for cancer in the past 6 months?

O Yes   O No

If you or your family have been diagnosed with colon polyps or cancer of any kind, what type(s), at what age(s) were they diagnosed, and are they living?

	Self		Mother		Father		Other	
	Yes	Age	Yes	Age	Yes	Age	Yes	Age
Breast Cancer	☐		☐		☐		☐	
Colon Polyps	☐		☐		☐		☐	
Colorectal Cancer	☐		☐		☐		☐	
Endometrial Cancer	☐		☐		☐		☐	
Gastric Cancer	☐		☐		☐		☐	
Pancreatic Cancer	☐		☐		☐		☐	
Ovarian Cancer	☐		☐		☐		☐	
Other	☐		☐		☐		☐	
Living?			O Yes		O Yes		O Yes	
			O No		O No		O No	

	Sister 1 Yes Age	**Sister 2** Yes Age	**Sister 3** Yes Age	**Sister 4** Yes Age
Breast Cancer	☐ ▢	☐ ▢	☐ ▢	☐ ▢
Colon Polyps	☐ ▢	☐ ▢	☐ ▢	☐ ▢
Colorectal Cancer	☐ ▢	☐ ▢	☐ ▢	☐ ▢
Endometrial Cancer	☐ ▢	☐ ▢	☐ ▢	☐ ▢
Gastric Cancer	☐ ▢	☐ ▢	☐ ▢	☐ ▢
Pancreatic Cancer	☐ ▢	☐ ▢	☐ ▢	☐ ▢
Ovarian Cancer	☐ ▢	☐ ▢	☐ ▢	☐ ▢
Other	☐ ▢	☐ ▢	☐ ▢	☐ ▢
Living?	O Yes O No	O Yes O No	O Yes O No	O Yes O No

	Brother 1 Yes Age	**Brother 2** Yes Age	**Brother 3** Yes Age	**Brother 4** Yes Age
Breast Cancer	☐ ▢	☐ ▢	☐ ▢	☐ ▢
Colon Polyps	☐ ▢	☐ ▢	☐ ▢	☐ ▢
Colorectal Cancer	☐ ▢	☐ ▢	☐ ▢	☐ ▢
Endometrial Cancer	☐ ▢	☐ ▢	☐ ▢	☐ ▢
Gastric Cancer	☐ ▢	☐ ▢	☐ ▢	☐ ▢
Pancreatic Cancer	☐ ▢	☐ ▢	☐ ▢	☐ ▢
Ovarian Cancer	☐ ▢	☐ ▢	☐ ▢	☐ ▢
Other	☐ ▢	☐ ▢	☐ ▢	☐ ▢
Living?	O Yes O No	O Yes O No	O Yes O No	O Yes O No

	Daughter 1		**Daughter 2**		**Son 1**		**Son 2**	
	Yes	Age	Yes	Age	Yes	Age	Yes	Age
Breast Cancer	☐		☐		☐		☐	
Colon Polyps	☐		☐		☐		☐	
Colorectal Cancer	☐		☐		☐		☐	
Endometrial Cancer	☐		☐		☐		☐	
Gastric Cancer	☐		☐		☐		☐	
Pancreatic Cancer	☐		☐		☐		☐	
Ovarian Cancer	☐		☐		☐		☐	
Other	☐		☐		☐		☐	
Living?	O Yes		O Yes		O Yes		O Yes	
	O No		O No		O No		O No	

	Maternal Aunt		**Maternal Uncle**		**Paternal Aunt**		**Paternal Uncle**	
	Yes	Age	Yes	Age	Yes	Age	Yes	Age
Breast Cancer	☐		☐		☐		☐	
Colon Polyps	☐		☐		☐		☐	
Colorectal Cancer	☐		☐		☐		☐	
Endometrial Cancer	☐		☐		☐		☐	
Gastric Cancer	☐		☐		☐		☐	
Pancreatic Cancer	☐		☐		☐		☐	
Ovarian Cancer	☐		☐		☐		☐	
Other	☐		☐		☐		☐	
Living?	O Yes		O Yes		O Yes		O Yes	
	O No		O No		O No		O No	

	Maternal ☐ Grandmother	Maternal ☐ Grandfather	Paternal ☐ Grandmother	Paternal Grandfather
	Yes ☐Age ☐	Yes ☐Age ☐	Yes ☐Age ☐	Yes ☐Age
Breast Cancer	☐	☐	☐	☐
Colon Polyps	☐	☐	☐	☐
Colorectal Cancer	☐	☐	☐	☐
Endometrial Cancer	☐	☐	☐	☐
Gastric Cancer	☐	☐	☐	☐
Pancreatic Cancer	☐	☐	☐	☐
Ovarian Cancer	☐	☐	☐	☐
Other	☐	☐	☐	☐
Living?	O Yes O No	O Yes O No	O Yes O No	O Yes O No

If you have any questions about this study, consent form, or survey please feel free to contact us:

Email: editors@oncolink.com
Tel.: (+01)-866-724-4100 (toll free)

Please mail your completed OncoLink/NCCRA survey and database consent form to:

OncoLink Editorial Office
University of Pennsylvania Cancer Center
3400 Spruce Street ☐ 2 Donner
Philadelphia
PA 19104
USA

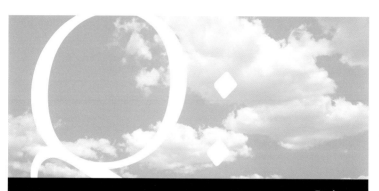

Index